CHILD
IS BORN

The Natural
Child Care Classic

WILHELM ZUR LINDEN, M.D.

Translated and edited by J. Collis

Healing Arts Press
Rochester, Vermont

Healing Arts Press
One Park Street
Rochester, Vermont 05767
www.InnerTraditions.com

*Note to the reader: This book is intended as an informational guide. The
remedies, approaches, and techniques described herein are meant to
supplement, and not to be a substitute for, professional medical care or
treatment. They should not be used to treat a serious ailment without
prior consultation with a qualified health-care professional.*

LIBRARY OF CONGRESS CATALOGING-IN-PUBLICATION DATA

Zur Linden, Wilhelm.
     When a child is born : the natural childcare classic /
Wilhelm zur Linden ; translated and edited by J. Collis.
               p.   cm.
     Includes index.
     ISBN 0-89281-751-8 (pbk. : alk. paper)
     1. Pregnancy. 2. Childbirth. 3. Infants—Care. 4. Child
care. 5. Child rearing. I. Collis, Johanna. II. Title.
RG525.Z874   1998   98-21689
649'.122—dc21   CIP

Printed and bound in Canada

10 9 8 7 6 5 4 3 2 1

Healing Arts Press is a division of Inner Traditions International

CONTENTS

Chapter Three
THE BIRTH

Chapter Four
THE POST-NATAL PERIOD

Chapter Five
THE BREAST-FEEDING PERIOD

Chapter Six
THE BABY IMMEDIATELY AFTER BIRTH

Chapter Seven
CARING FOR THE BABY

Chapter Eight
FEEDING THE BABY

Chapter Nine
SOME GENERAL POINTS ABOUT FEEDING CHILDREN

Chapter Ten
UPBRINGING

Chapter Eleven
THE SICK CHILD

Contents

7

FOREWORD

Dr. Wilhelm zur Linden's book *When a Child Is Born* has often been referred to as a "bible" for mothers and fathers. Since its first printing in Germany in 1957 it has helped generations of parents during pregnancy and labor and in understanding infancy and early childhood in all its complexity. Above all, the book is an invaluable reference for dealing with children's illnesses. It appeared in English in 1984 and has become a classic here as well.

Dr. zur Linden's approach to human biology in its very early phase is based on Rudolph Steiner's Anthroposophy. In the beginning of the twentieth century this Austrian philosopher described the human being's threefold nature—body, soul, and spirit, as well as the threefoldedness of thinking, feeling, and willing, which forms the basis of our higher nature. To be born, for Steiner, means to incarnate gradually into this threefoldedness. Whatever happens during all phases of life, from infancy to old age, relates in different kinds of ways to all three aspects of the human being.

Steiner's holistic philosophy calls for a very conscious approach to education and healing. Consequently, Steiner founded a school in 1919 (the first Waldorf School, in Stuttgart) and several hospitals. He also laid the basis for a different kind of medicine, which today is produced by the Weleda and Wala pharmaceutical companies. Both the medical and the educational impulse have grown tremendously in the last seventy years. Meanwhile there is a considerable number of anthroposophical hospitals. Worldwide, more than seven hundred schools are established all over the world.

When a Child Is Born helps us to understand the process of pregnancy, birth, infancy, and early childhood as the incarnation of a spiritual individuality, who meets numerous obstacles by connecting to a physical body. From the growing embryo in the womb to caring for the baby in the cradle and raising the child until the child is a preschooler, the book tells the reader in short and clearly outlined chapters what to do.

Dr. zur Linden gives concrete advice on how to feed the baby during different ages and includes suggestions in the case of special dietary needs.

For many readers, the chapter "The Sick Child" is reason enough to buy the book. The author explains the physical, psychological, and spiritual aspects of different illnesses during childhood. His special focus on the meaning of illness is very important for our Western culture because it gives us the opportunity to see illness from a very different viewpoint. Allopathic medicine offers a wide and helpful arsenal of remedies for which we can surely be thankful, but Dr. zur Linden asks us to look beyond and to understand illness and its treatment in a spiritual as well as a physical way.

Already before the birth of a child we adults find ourselves puzzled and sometimes helpless. The question of how we can face the upcoming challenges often becomes an existential one. The whole life of the family changes all of a sudden—nothing is as it was before. Parents as well as children face a never-ending learning process. The family as the primary social nucleus is the earliest learning group, growing together through different crises and joys. In this network of interrelation the complex path of growing up takes place. And as we approach the end of the century, the upbringing of children is more than ever an activity that requires preparation, study, and a lot of thinking.

Why is it so important that *When a Child Is Born* comes to the reader in a new edition for the twenty-first century? The place and the role of the child in our society have changed dramatically. It is no exaggeration to say that infancy, childhood, and adolescence are under attack by social, economic, and environmental threats. Advertisements and media usurp the role of educators and more often than not act as manipulators. Social changes are equally immense: the role of parents is constantly being defined anew. Finally, environmental changes threaten our children. Pollution in its many aspects often makes it impossible for children to experience nature in its purity. The implications of these threats are not considered closely enough.

The incarnation of a human being is a complex process that requires as much help as possible. *When a Child Is Born* can be of immense value in this endeavor. This pragmatic, practical, and spiritual guide offers that rarest of combinations—quick advice and profound insight.

Hans-Joachim Mattke

INTRODUCTION

The source of life

Even in the biggest cities, when the sprouting and budding of spring begins, we cannot fail to notice how an abundance of leaf and plant substance that was not there before comes into being. Naturally the leaves come out of the branches of the tree and the plants out of the seeds, yet the minutest inspection with the most powerful microscope cannot reveal why in the course of time a plant or an enormous tree should arise from a tiny seed.

But we need no instruments to tell us that this process cannot take place without certain conditions, namely the warmth of spring and summer and above all water and light. If these influences are removed, that is if it is cold, dry and dark, no growth can possibly occur. That is why we create these conditions in order to prevent life or further growth. For instance we preserve foodstuffs in cold, dark and dry conditions.

The origin of the forces that create and carry life are found in sunlight, which is also the source of the earth's warmth, in air and in water.

We see therefore that the essential element is not the material, which was already present in a dead form. That a living substance can arise out of the dead matter depends above all upon the influence of light. Light and other cosmic forces are the source of all life. A time will come when these cosmic forces are the object of scientific research, just as is the case today with matter. Meanwhile, however, in our understandable and natural eagerness to penetrate the world of matter, we have forgotten and neglected the cosmic forces and influences. Without these formative forces from the cosmos, mediated above all through water, neither plant, nor animal, nor man could come into being or live.

The origin of man

So life does not sprout out of the seed or ovum. No one believes any longer that the life for generations of plants or animals is packed into a single seed. Instead we see the seed or ovum as the point into which the life forces from the cosmos can flow, for they cannot work their way into dead matter.

It is quite untrue, though still often stated, that a simple form of life gradually evolved into more complicated forms over aeons of time, leading finally to the immense complexity of man, the 'crown of creation'. Just as a living substance cannot develop out of dead matter, so man, a spiritual being, cannot develop out of living substance alone.

We have seen that cosmic forces are needed to create life. Similarly spiritual forces must flow into a living human ovum if a spirit is to live in it. These forces are not electric impulses or cosmic rays but spiritual influences filled with the greatest wisdom. They were present at the beginning of creation. The powers of creation are quite real and are described in the Bible and all the world's mythologies.

Our forefathers were surely closer to the truth than we are today when their great leaders in pre-Christian times spoke of the existence and working of intelligent spiritual beings whose task it was to care for the welfare of every human being. Measured against the whole of human history it is only quite recently, since natural scientific thinking began to take hold, that we have come to believe that human life and growth can be explained solely in relation to the chemical and physical laws of matter.

The early Christians in their wisdom described the spiritual beings who were more exalted than man quite matter of factly as angels, archangels and so on. They are the helpers of the divine Creator in the making and preserving of the universe and man.

The physical part of man is very well-known today, too well-known perhaps, so that the spirit behind it is no longer seen. The embryo in the womb grows from a fertilised ovum which is embedded in the wall of the womb much as a plant seed is embedded in the earth. Growth is nourished by the motherly 'soil', the mother's blood and life forces which the embryo quite inconsiderately draws towards itself. Growth at this level can, however, at best be seen as a kind of life resembling that of a plant. But to regard a man as no more than a biological being is nonsensical. As such he would have no life task and no justification for existence in the world. To seek the origin of man's soul and spirit in this way would be the equivalent of a technician making a chemical analysis of a radio or gramophone record in order to discover the music he can obtain from them. Though the music cannot reach him without this medium, yet by its nature it is totally different. In the same way the 'biological being' is only the bearer of the spirit and the soul.

While the plant is indeed a purely biological being, an animal, in addition to its biological body, also has a soul. This lives in the animal, enabling it to express joy and sorrow, feelings which are non-existent for the plant. The animal is able to possess a soul because its body is quite different from that of the plant. It is not the body that creates the soul, but the soul needs a living organism that differs greatly from that of a plant.

The difference between animal and man is as great as that between plant and animal. The most obvious distinction between a higher mammal and the human being is that the animal at or shortly after birth possesses all the capabilities it needs for life. Man, on the other hand, has to master his capabilities by slow degrees, whereby to become a true human being is the hardest battle of all. The animal is virtually complete at birth and only grows in size and strength up to the point when it is able to reproduce its kind. After this, nothing really new is added.

At birth the human being is unfinished, helpless and incapable of maintaining life or even moving from place to place. Compared with a young animal a human baby is born prematurely. In saying 'The more noble and perfect a thing, the longer it needs before achieving completion', Schopenhauer described an essential characteristic of human development. In this context perfection does not refer to a physical state of affairs. All organs and physical capabilities are far more perfectly developed in animals than in man. The animal's legs are stronger and it can run, jump and swim faster and better than man. Its legs are specialised for this. Thanks to its quite different 'perfection', however, the human hand is not at all specialised, and so the human being can do 'anything' with it.

This alone should be enough to show clearly that animals cannot be the ancestors of man, for a specialisation can only develop from something that is unspecialised. Thus man has not descended from the ape but the apes and other higher mammals are instead 'relations' that man has left behind in the course of his development. This is why a new-born monkey looks so human, in the shape of its head particularly, and it is also why the resemblance fades as the monkey grows up. If man were descended from the ape, then a new-born baby would resemble an ape, an absurd and grotesque notion.

The human being is 'the firstborn of creation'. The purpose of creation is the human being, and by remaining behind at a lower level the animals, through a kind of sacrifice, have enabled him to develop.

How does the spirit of man differ from the soul, which is also possessed by animals? The simplest and yet also the most characteristic manifestation of the human being is his upright posture and gait, his speaking, and his thinking.

No animal standing or walking on two legs is in fact upright. For man, on the other hand, the only worthy posture is upright, and it is not for nothing that when we speak of an 'upright person' we mean his character.

That human speech differs fundamentally from the

sign language of animals is hardly noticed today because there is little understanding for the true nature of speech. It is seen as no more than a means of communication when in reality it is wisdom-filled and closely linked with the process of creation.

Through speech the child learns to think. Unfortunately thinking is today seen as something merely intellectual that can be measured by tests. In its origin it is far greater than this. Even the most sophisticated intelligence tests cannot encompass anything to do with real wisdom. Similarly a wise deed or wise counsel can, on occasion, be understood by an intelligent person as something stupid. This is why it is so important to develop all the spiritual capacities of children instead of one-sidedly training their intelligence.

The ego of man

All living creatures endowed with feeling and consciousness, that is animals and human beings, have a soul. But in the soul there is a centre possessed by man alone. This is the human spirit, the divine spark that uses the soul and body as an instrument in accordance with its own character. As this spiritual spark distinguishes the individual from all his fellow men, it can also be called the 'I' or ego.

This is the inmost kernel of our being, it is the essential unique personality we meet in every individual.

We cannot examine closely enough the difference between man and animal. A wild animal is innocent of any excess or vice. Man, on the other hand, knows these only too well, and increasingly, as he develops away from nature towards a civilisation that is remote from life. Animals never overeat or indulge in excesses. Especially their sexual life runs its course in an almost ascetically orderly fashion under rigid temporal controls.

We might, then, be tempted to say that the animal leads a more moral life than man. This is a considerable, though frequent, error. The animal is bound by the laws that regulate its own life and that of its environment. Man is the only creature with the freedom to say 'no'. His brain can encompass every conceivable thought, his hand grasp at everything, his heart long for everything and his will desire everything. He is not as bound by natural laws as the animal; to a large degree he can act freely because he has an ego. This ego is the unique part of the human being and it is this that builds for itself an individual body. At birth it begins to take possession of this body. Of course the unborn embryo in the womb is alive and it can thus not be said that human life begins at birth. But at birth the ego of the human being unites with the body. Many years pass, however, before the body born of the mother is entirely permeated by the child's ego, for the ego must first transform and exchange every part of the inherited living substance in order to build its own individual body. The exchange of substance continues throughout life, for man continues to transform himself.

The process by which the ego unites with the body is called incarnation.

Where does this spiritual ego, which unites with the body at birth, come from? And what is the situation of the embryo before birth?

Describing the mystery of birth in olden times, the leaders of mankind used to speak of the stork who brought the babies. Since children in those days were born to mothers in much the same way as they are today, this picture cannot be taken to refer to the birth of the body, especially as there was no secret about this. The fairy tales of all cultured peoples speak of the assistance given to mankind by white birds such as swans, doves and storks. These white birds are a pictorial description of beings who create a link between the spiritual and the earthly world. So in the stork we have a picture of the ego of man being carried from heaven to earth. For our forefathers this was obviously the decisive process, more important than the physical and physiological process of birth, for the spirit was more important for them than the body.

At birth the ego incarnates in the body. At the moment of death it lays aside the body and is free once more, while the body disintegrates. The indestructible ego lives on in the spiritual world, the home from which it emerged for a while to live on the earth. This path of the spirit after death is still a certainty in varying degrees for many people of our time. But what humanity as a whole has largely forgotten today is that after a long journey through the spiritual world the ego returns, perhaps after several centuries, to incarnate once more in a new body conceived by new parents. This process is termed 'reincarnation'. All the great cultures of the world have known about this and the Bible speaks of it in several places. More recently, enlightened individuals such as Goethe and Lessing and many others have been quite convinced of the reality of this process. But on the whole this knowledge has been lost for several centuries in the Western world. This has been necessary for the progress of mankind, but now Rudolf Steiner's Anthroposophy has made this knowledge available once more for modern man.

Those who feel these ideas to be totally alien to them should certainly not attempt to 'believe' them. It is better to inform oneself in more detail and then attempt to live with the ideas for a while. Sickness, fate and death, indeed the whole of man's life, acquire new meaning. Questions arising from the death of a child or from some other blow of fate, questions raised when a 'bad' man is favoured by fortune while a 'good' one meets with endless ill luck, cannot be answered without a view of these relatively short spaces of time on earth as part of a much longer process in which a person may in a later life compensate for the failings of an earlier one. An abundance of questions and answers present themselves at the idea that the spiritual kernel, the ego of every individual, not only continues to exist in a new way after death but also one day returns for a new life on earth.

This picture of the child coming down to us is the basis for the reverence with which we should approach him. If we have this inner attitude we shall never make the common mistake of many parents who regard their children as their property or even as a toy. In addition we shall not be in danger of imagining that we are capable of creating our children. Of course without the uniting of a man and a woman and without the availability of a womb no child will be born; but the parents are no more than helpers in this marvellous event of the joining of a spiritual being with an earthly body formed by an act of divine creation and placed at that spirit's command for a whole lifetime.

Chapter One

THE GROWING EMBRYO

Expecting the child

Fortunately most women when they discover they are pregnant are far more delighted with the prospect than alarmed at the mysterious process now going on within their body. But even so, lack of knowledge or faulty information often lead to anxiety and may be the source of some of the problems of pregnancy. This book is intended to provide the answers to many questions about pregnancy, birth and diet, and care of the infant and small child.

Signs of pregnancy

Women who menstruate regularly can be fairly sure they are pregnant if a monthly period fails to occur, and if the following period also fails to appear, a pregnancy is virtually certain. With healthy women whose menstruation is irregular, the missing of one or several periods is not a sure sign of pregnancy. They should consult their doctor about possible blood or urine tests which can give early certainty, or purchase a test kit at the chemist. The doctor can also determine a pregnancy of six weeks or more by internal examination.

Further signs, in addition to the cessation of menstruation, are enlargement of the breasts, their secretion of small amounts of colostrum (a yellowish fluid which precedes the formation of milk after the baby is born), morning nausea or sickness, frequent urge to pass water, and excessive weariness in the evening. Some women, however, feel particularly healthy and vigorous when pregnant and do not suffer from tiredness or nausea.

The final and unmistakable signs of pregnancy do not occur till the fifth month, when the mother feels the baby's movements for the first time and when the doctor can hear the baby's heartbeat with his stethoscope and feel the different parts of the embryo.

Expected date of birth

To calculate the probable date of the baby's birth, women with a normal menstrual cycle of 28 days should take the first day of their last period, subtract three months and add seven days. This will give the date in the following year when the baby may be expected. For example: Last regular period started 5th November; three months earlier 5th August; add seven days and the probable date of birth will be 12th August in the following year.

However, this rule of thumb must be taken as a very rough guide only, since every child has his own, for him normal, needs which determine the length of pregnancy. The average is 280 to 282 days or ten lunar months, though one usually speaks of nine calendar months or forty weeks.

The baby's movements can first be felt almost exactly in the middle of a first pregnancy. In a second or subsequent pregnancy the movements are felt 12 to 14 days earlier.

Life conditions in the womb

On the one hand the embryo is in a most wonderful way embedded in the mother's womb which gives it perfect protection. On the other hand it is separated from the mother's organism by the walls of the womb and the foetal membranes. These membranes are extremely important for the developing child because as the embryo grows they play a part in the gradual uniting of the child's soul and spirit with the body. At birth their task is complete and they are then discarded as 'afterbirth'. The work of the placenta is similar. This is an organ filled with the mother's blood and it serves to nourish the child. At the same time it serves as a filter, so that the stream of nourishment does not flow direct from the mother's organism to the embryo.

Thus the embryo is carried, protected and nourished by the mother, and yet its development and growth takes place for the most part quite separately from the mother's organism. The membranes and placenta in many ways isolate it from the life of the mother.

Other remarkable conditions also surround the embryo. Floating in the waters of the womb, it is hardly subject to the force of gravity. Furthermore it contains an extremely small proportion of firm mineral substance: At 3 to 4 months the embryo consists of 93 per cent water, and even at birth it is still 80 per cent fluid. Thus only about one fifth of the little body is solid matter. The embryo also lives and grows in the womb with a very small amount of oxygen, which in turn affects the number of red blood corpuscles and the amount of haemoglobin.

Chapter Two

PREGNANCY

Medical examination during pregnancy

The expectant mother should see her gynaecologist for an examination after the sixth week of pregnancy. He will want to check her blood pressure, blood count (possible anaemia) and kidney activity and also ascertain that her pelvis will allow the baby to pass through the birth canal. (For instance, a malformed pelvis, possibly due to rickets, could present an obstacle.)

Even if the first examination is satisfactory, the mother should see the gynaecologist regularly throughout the pregnancy. She should inform him about illnesses in the family such as epilepsy or diabetes and also about any acute feverish illnesses she may have had. He must be notified of any bleeding from the vagina immediately, even if it seems insignificant. Regarding the *rhesus factor* see page 32 and regarding *vaccination* during pregnancy see pages 29 and 169.

Ailments of pregnancy

Pregnancy can be the cause of trivial and sometimes also more serious ailments, especially if the expectant mother is in some way unable to adjust to her new situation or cope with the greater demands made on her. Quite independently from this, however, a mother may be plagued by discomforts in her first pregnancy and free of them during the second, and vice versa.

Morning nausea or sickness, when only gastric juices and hardly ever food are brought up, does not lead to loss of weight. Relief can often be achieved by chewing some raw oat flakes. It is also helpful to drink two to three cups of Weleda Pinella tea (or any other herbal tea specified for liver and gall) daily. Sometimes, however, there is serious and prolonged vomiting of the food eaten. In these cases the doctor should be consulted, since there is usually also lack of appetite, and considerable weight loss can ensue. Great care must be taken to correct resulting deficiencies in mineral salts (iron, calcium) and vitamins.

For *heartburn* it is helpful to take Weleda Digestodoron (20 drops 3 times daily). Alternatively one can chew a few hazel or cashew nuts till they become a tasteless pulp in the mouth. When this is swallowed it controls the gastric acids.

Excessive flow of saliva plagues some expectant mothers, sometimes more than a litre (two pints) a day. This can often be improved by chewing a few dried juniper berries very well.

Swellings on face or legs should definitely be shown to the doctor (take a sample of early morning urine). If he finds the cause to be merely congestion, Weleda Skin Tone Lotion rubbed into the skin is a good remedy.

Excessive tiredness can frequently be caused by anaemia, and should therefore be investigated. It is wrong, however, to take any iron preparation without first undergoing a blood test. The same applies to other medicines, vitamin preparations, etc. Synthetic vitamin D in any form should be avoided. If anaemia is diagnosed, it should be treated immediately. This is also important in the case of any circulatory weakness.

Difficulty in breathing, particularly during the last three months, can be caused by the increasing lack of space in the abdomen. It is a help to breathe calmly and deeply in and out (particularly out!).

Palpitations (which sometimes accompany breathlessness) and *pains in the sciatic nerve* do not usually require any special treatment.

Congestion of blood in the veins of the legs, which causes *varicose veins,* should be treated. Apart from taking certain medicines for the circulation, it is often a help to bandage the legs with elastic bandages or to wear support stockings.

Constipation must definitely be avoided. The following is a useful recipe: In the evening, soak in half a pint (quarter of a litre) of cold water one dessert spoon each of wheat bran, wheat germ and whole linseed together with one or two chopped figs or prunes. Eat this either cold or heated for breakfast the next morning.

Depressive moods and even thoughts of suicide, also rapid changes of mood, belong to the difficulties experienced by some women in pregnancy. They are rarely serious and usually pass without treatment. The same goes for unusual *cravings* for certain foods and acute *dislike* of others.

Piles and *varicose vulva* are difficulties experienced frequently in pregnancy and can cause the expectant mother great discomfort, quite overshadowing the happy mood which should prevail during her time of waiting. Women who remain at work well into pregnancy are particularly prone to these afflictions, which are caused by circulatory congestion in the abdomen. The doctor can and must help. In less serious cases Weleda Stibium 0.4% Suppositories for piles are helpful. They contain a remedy which stimulates the circulation. A daily and easy movement of the bowels is also essential (see recipe above). It can also be helpful to sit in a cold bath for six seconds (not longer!) every evening, after which one wraps the lower part of the body in a Turkish towel and goes to bed without drying.

Stretch marks appear on the mother's abdomen, and sometimes even on breasts and thighs, as her girth increases. These can remain visible after the birth of the baby and should be rubbed with a good skin oil.

Patches like freckles can appear on the mother's face, but these disappear on their own after the birth of the baby.

Threats to the embryo

Among the most frequent causes of malformation are abortion attempts, either with instruments or by chemical means.

With some virus infections (especially German measles, but also mumps, chicken pox and Asian flu) there is a danger that the virus might pass from the mother's to the child's blood. If this happens, malformations are especially likely in the first three months. The same applies to smallpox vaccination (see page 169), which should therefore be avoided during pregnancy, especially during the first three and in the final months. Live oral vaccination against polio should also be avoided, particularly during the early months. Treatment with BCG vaccine against tuberculosis is only recommended if the expectant mother has unavoidable close contact with a patient suffering from open tuberculosis where isolation is impossible.

The thalidomide tragedy has shown the dangers of sleeping pills. And of course thalidomide is not the only substance that can cripple the embryo. Doctors all over the world agree that the unchecked use of pills of all kinds constitutes an increasing threat to mankind, and this threat is magnified in pregnancy.

Large doses of hormones, for instance cortisone, taken during the first three months of pregnancy, have been shown to cause serious malformations such as cleft lip and cleft palate.

An expectant mother must not be allowed to undergo any kind of X-ray examination or treatment on any part of the body except in life or death situations. The same applies of course to radio-therapy of all kinds.

There are a number of other diseases and environmental causes that can damage the embryo. Among these are venereal diseases and certain parasites such as canine tape-worms. Shocks should be avoided. An unbalanced and qualitatively inferior diet can have undesirable consequences. Radioactive contamination of food and drinking water is an environmental threat of which the consequences for future generations cannot as yet be accurately foreseen.

Morning sickness does not on the whole affect the embryo, but babies whose mothers have experienced serious sickness during pregnancy should be carefully examined and kept under observation for several years by their doctor.

Smoking during pregnancy and the period of breast feeding

Since smoking is still on the increase, the subject cannot be omitted from a book of this kind.

There should certainly be no smoking when babies and small children are in the room. It has been shown that the pulse of an unborn child accelerates after only a few inhalations by the mother, and nursing mothers can even cause nicotine poisoning in their babies, for nicotine is one of the strongest poisons known to us.

Recent research has shown that the amount of vitamin C in the milk of smoking mothers is considerably lower than in that of mothers who do not smoke. It was found in addition that this lack of vitamin C could not be corrected by the consumption of either additional citrus fruit or vitamin C tablets. This is another way in which smoking by expectant and nursing mothers damages the child, for the baby needs a great deal of vitamin C, especially in winter and spring.

Many smokers repeatedly attempt to break this habit. An expectant or nursing mother is responsible not only for herself but also for a growing human being, her child. There is only one effective measure with which to combat addiction to nicotine: Give up smoking today.

Toxoplasmosis

A minute parasite in the mother's blood penetrates the placenta and invades the blood of the embryo, which either dies or, less frequently, suffers severe damage mainly to the nervous system, in which inflammation is generated. Usually severe and as yet irreversible damage is done to the brain, eyes or ears.

The parasites are transferred to the mother from domestic animals, dogs, cats, rabbits, sheep, pigeons and animals bred for their fur. Pregnant women who have contact with these creatures should be examined even if they themselves do not feel ill. Early treatment can prevent damage to the child.

This illness is becoming more frequent and it is advisable to undergo a blood test before contemplating pregnancy.

The rhesus factor

Research using the blood of rhesus monkeys has revealed that many miscarriages are connected with certain characteristics of the red blood corpuscles. The blood of about 85% of the population is 'rhesus positive', while that of the remainder is 'rhesus negative'. If both parents are the same, either positive or negative, or if the mother is rhesus positive and the father rhesus negative, there is nothing to worry about.

But if the father is rhesus positive and the mother rhesus negative there may be trouble, namely if the baby inherits the father's positive factor. In such cases it is possible for some of the baby's rhesus positive blood to enter the mother's bloodstream via the placenta, whereupon her system will start to make antibodies to combat the 'foreign' blood, either during the pregnancy or after the birth. Though this does not usually affect the first child, subsequent children can be seriously harmed: the destruction of the red blood corpuscles leads to acute anaemia, or a fatal attack of jaundice immediately after birth, or severe brain damage.

These babies can be saved by a complete exchange of blood within six hours of birth, a method which has so far shown no damaging side effects.

Parents who are in this difficult position can take certain steps to minimise the situation. The mother herself should avoid having blood transfusions if at all possible, but in an emergency the blood she is given must be carefully selected taking into account not only her blood group but also the rhesus factor. It is feared that even fairly frequent intramuscular injections of blood can sensitise the recipient's blood, so in these cases, too, the rhesus factor must be taken into account. (The whole problem has nothing to do with ordinary blood groups.)

The mother should eat plenty of citrus fruit which has a high vitamin C content and should take care that her calcium count is sufficiently high (but not by taking vitamin D!). These two factors will help reduce the brittleness of the tiny blood vessels, thus helping to prevent any of the child's blood from escaping through the placenta into her blood stream.

There is now also an anti-rhesus serum which is injected into the mother immediately after the birth as a protection for a future child.

Avoiding miscarriage

During the first three months and from the seventh month of pregnancy miscarriages or premature births are not too unusual, particularly in the case of a first pregnancy or when there has been a previous miscarriage. During the other months miscarriage is also possible, but less likely.

As a normal precaution one should avoid heavy carrying, lifting or stretching (e.g. hanging up washing) and also squatting for any length of time. Long rides in buses or cars and any riding on motor cycles should be avoided because of the shaking and jarring these cause.

The expectant mother should have plenty of rest, going to bed early and lying down for one or two hours after lunch. She should undress and relax completely in bed.

Strong laxatives are to be avoided and constipation treated by adhering to the right diet taken with sufficient water. Laxative teas are also useful, for example Weleda Clairo Tea taken not too strong. See also the recipe mentioned in the section on *Ailments of pregnancy*.

The danger to the child if the mother smokes during pregnancy is discussed on page 31.

If there is any danger of a miscarriage, marital intercourse should be avoided, particularly when the monthly periods would be due.

Any movement which disturbs the natural rhythms of the organism is unfavourable, for instance typing, sewing by machine and many other machine jobs, if they have to be carried out for hours on end.

Occupations which require sitting with the upper part of the body bent forward are also unsuitable.

During pregnancy one should not totally immerse oneself in any activity, even such household chores as stirring, winding wool or knitting. The many-sided activity of the housewife is really the most suited to pregnancy so long as nothing is overdone. But the housewife should not think that her work in the house or even her walks to the shops can be a substitute for regular carefree walks when she tries to let nothing weigh on her mind.

Signs of danger

Pregnant women are safeguarded against many dangers as though they were under a special mantle of protection. On the whole they do not succumb to ordinary illnesses and the majority feel particularly well, better than at any other time in their lives. They are fitter, more balanced and more resistant to infection and illness.

It is therefore more as a cautionary measure and for reassurance that a number of symptoms are listed below about which the doctor should be consulted without delay. (It is practical to take a sample of early morning urine with you straight away):

- bleeding resembling that of the monthly period even if less profuse. If this occurs one should go straight to bed and lie on one's back, keeping the legs quite still, until the doctor arrives.
- excessive nausea and vomiting after the third month and serious faintness;

- swelling of hands, ankles and eyelids;
- weight increases of more than two pounds (one kilogram) per month.

Sport during pregnancy

The best 'sport' during pregnancy is the mother's regular daily walk, but she should remember that in the later months a quarter of an hour's physical activity is equivalent to an hour when not pregnant. Swimming can also be encouraged during the first half of pregnancy if the water is not too cold or the waves too high. But the expectant mother should not dive or swim under water.

It is best to avoid eurythmy, gymnastics, ski-ing, tennis, athletics, and anything else which requires strenuous muscular exertion or jarring of the body. If possible the mother should not subject herself to extreme changes of altitude, whether by travelling from low-lying parts into high mountains or vice versa, or by flying.

As the baby grows, the mother will find her breathing becoming increasingly shallow and she might feel short of breath. A simple breathing exercise can be helpful. Stand by an open window wearing a loose dress. Breathe in and out through the nose, taking care particularly to empty the lungs completely on the out-breath. Do not, however, pause before breathing in again, nor before breathing out when the lungs are quite filled. Raise the arms lightly on the in-breath and lower them on the out-breath. Ten long breaths like this three times daily should suffice.

The doctor will advise on special gymnastics suitable for pregnancy. The most important thing is to avoid excesses of any kind.

Diet during pregnancy

Those who anyway have a varied diet of good quality food need not change their ways much when pregnant. Within reason one can eat what one pleases and even yield to any cravings one might suddenly have. It is important to have regular meals and better to add an extra meal rather than eat too much at a time.

The expectant mother should be very careful about the amount of tea and coffee she drinks. The same applies to maté tea which contains a considerable amount of caffeine. The soft drinks now on the market which contain caffeine are also unsuitable. In addition to caffeine they contain a number of undesirable chemicals, the most dubious being orthophosphoric acid, which provides the stimulating effect. This acid can damage the liver, particularly as the advertisements advise that these drinks should be taken ice cold. Alcohol and smoking are out of the question during pregnancy. Hot spices also should not be used.

Our diet these days usually contains too much protein, so the expectant mother should take eggs, meat and fish in small quantities only. An egg a day is absolute nonsense, and anyway eggs which are more than eight or ten days old have lost much of their nutritional value. The meat eaten should where possible be that of young animals.

When changing to a vegetarian diet, care must be

taken to ensure that deficiencies, especially of protein, do not arise. Normal protein needs can be met with curd cheese (see recipe page 209), cottage cheese, milk and cereals. Vegetables should be as free as possible of chemical additives and other impurities and vegetables that cause flatulence (such as cabbage and dried pulses) should be avoided.

As a general guide it can be said that during the first three months Bircher muesli and sour fruits are excellent foods, whereas too many pastry and farinaceous dishes should be avoided.

During the second three-month period sweet fruits, particularly from southern countries (including almonds), are specially desirable.

And during the last three months all kinds of cereals are good because of their mineral content (wheat barley, green rye, millet; and oats to a lesser extent).

The daily food of an expectant mother should include: high-quality dark rye bread, at least half a pint (quarter of a litre) of milk daily in any form (including yogurt, sour milk, butter milk, kefir), fresh vegetables, every kind of salad (e.g. lettuce, lamb's lettuce, endive, cress, cucumber), fruit in season, and fresh herbs daily if possible (parsley, chives, sweet basil, savory, fennel, lovage, thyme, marjoram) or powdered if not available fresh. They can be grown in the kitchen in flower pots if necessary.

Recent research (G.A. Winter and others) suggests that it is the substances and forces discovered in herbs such as these which gave our parents and grand-parents their greater resistance to infections of various kinds, so our present-day proclivity to infections of all sorts is reason enough to pay more attention once again to these herbs.

It is often believed in error that plenty of fruit can be a substitute for vegetables. But vegetables contain indispensable mineral salts which are not found in fruit.

Regular bowel habits go hand in hand with the right dietary habits. The right kind of bread is a particular help here and many suitable breads can be obtained in delicatessen and health food shops, for instance lactose bread, Waerland bread, Demeter bread, Steinmetz bread, Felke bread, pumpernickel, dark breads baked in wood ovens. Bread should not be eaten too fresh. Kollath Wheat Flakes, obtainable in health food shops, are also good.

Constipation can also arise as a result of too little fluid being taken. Herb teas, fruit juices and elixirs (Sandthorn, Rose Hip, Blackthorn, etc.) should be taken instead of milk, which can often cause constipation and flatulence.

Care of teeth for mother and child

It is often said that every child costs the mother a tooth. This is quite untrue if the right precautions are taken, even though the child does need a great deal of calcium and other salts. It is, however, a mistake to imagine that calcium or vitamin tablets can help. In the milk, cheese, bread, vegetables and even often the drinking water of a healthy diet there is more calcium than is required daily by the human organism. It is the ability to absorb the calcium which is disturbed in many people and which leads to a calcium deficiency in the blood. Then the calcium taken in tablet form is excreted along with the calcium in the daily food. Thus the greater need for calcium that arises through pregnancy remains unsatisfied. The expectant mother's saliva lacks the ability to protect the teeth from the acids arising in her mouth from bacterial activity in remnants of food.

Calcium taken in homoeopathic doses gradually stimulates the impaired ability to absorb calcium, so that the organism can learn once again to take in the necessary amounts for mother and baby from the food eaten. Many doctors find Weleda Calcium Supplements I and II particularly effective.

Essential for proper care of the teeth is a small toothbrush that can reach even the awkward crevices. Nylon bristles are preferred, as natural bristle collects bacteria too easily. The toothpaste used should not contain chemical disinfectants. Recommended are Weleda dental creams and saline paste.

Preparing physically for the birth of the baby

Pregnancy is not an illness, indeed often it is a time of enhanced physical well-being. Those who already live sensibly and healthily need not make many changes in their way of life.

Care of the skin is important during pregnancy. Weleda Skin Tone Lotion is stimulating and refreshing and can be used daily: Brushing with a dry brush or loofah also stimulates the circulation in the right way.

Women should not take warm baths more than twice

a week and during pregnancy these should not be warmer than 97°F (36°C). Weleda Pine and Lavender bath milks may be added.

During the ninth month one can prepare for the birth by taking a hipbath with lime blossom tea every other day: Pour two pints (1 litre) of boiling water on to a handful of lime blossoms, cover and allow to infuse for five minutes and then strain. Add this to the hipbath, which should not be hotter than 99°F (37°C). Stay in the bath for about ten minutes at first, but during the last two weeks for five minutes only.

Sunbathing should be undertaken with extreme caution and never for long periods at a time. Use a good herbal lotion for protecting the skin.

Early care of the nipples is important. If they are rather flat they should be drawn out gently night and morning. A milk pump can be used for this if they are too flat. Unsuitable non-porous brassieres often damage the nipples and cause them to loose their natural firmness. During the later months of pregnancy they should be rubbed daily with a few drops of lemon juice to help them regain their proper firmness. Oil or a greasy cream should only be used occasionally, otherwise the surface becomes too flabby.

The breasts themselves also lose their firmness when brassieres are too tight. A brief daily massage, rubbing from the base to the nipple, will help strengthen them and they should now be allowed to develop freely so that they will not lose shape through breast-feeding.

The importance of regular bowel habits in preparation for the baby's birth has already been discussed. This can be achieved with the right diet (see page 28 and 34).

Expectant mothers usually have a great need for sleep and should have ten hours at night and at least one hour in the middle of the day, when they should undress and go to bed properly.

Daily walks in the fresh air have already been mentioned.

Marital intercourse can do no harm until about eight weeks before the birth is expected, but should be strictly avoided if there is any danger of a miscarriage.

It is unwise during pregnancy to submit to any great changes in altitude, for instance holidays in the mountains if one lives in a lowland area. Flying is also best avoided.

When sitting, the legs should not be crossed, as this considerably impairs the circulation.

Psychological preparation for the baby's arrival

It is essential during the whole of pregnancy to practise what might be called soul hygiene. The baby cannot flourish if the mother's soul is filled with worry and anxiety (don't listen to old wives' tales of woe), but he thrives if she is filled with calm happiness and anticipation. A depressed mood causes cramped breathing, which in turn leads to many organic disturbances.

Particularly important is the avoidance of shocks of any kind. Cinema and television are thus unsuitable entertainment during pregnancy, since any moment something might be shown which could cause an unexpected shock.

Pregnancy is not a time for seeking diversions but rather a period of life which calls for an inner concentration of all one's soul forces on the happy event which is soon to take place. As a help in this inner collecting of thoughts and feelings, Rudolf Steiner often suggested that expectant mothers might contemplate a beautiful picture. He particularly recommended the Madonna pictures by Raphael, above all the Sistine Madonna. Contemplating this in peace and feeling its content in her soul, the mother will soon discover the helpful strength such a picture can give.

I do not mean that the mother should burden her soul with all sorts of weighty problems. But to ponder seriously on the fundamental questions of life and also her responsibility towards the child she is expecting need not darken her basic mood of joyous expectation.

Preparing older siblings for the arrival

It is important to speak to the other children in the family about the expected baby as early as possible and they may like to feel the baby moving inside 'mummy's tummy'. It is also right to tell them the old tale of the stork who brings down the child's soul from heaven. This will not contradict for them the fact of the baby growing inside their mother's body, for children have a natural understanding of the truths which in ancient times wise men clothed in pictures like that of the stork.

If told about the expected baby in the right way, the older children are sure to share in the happy expectation and they will do their best to be good when they know that their mother is carrying the child. It is indeed their right to share in the preparations, for after all, the new arrival will be their own brother or sister, theirs to protect and look after.

In the case of a home confinement it is best to send the older children away for a few days if possible, but as soon as they return they should not be neglected, otherwise they may become jealous. They should be allowed to participate in and watch everything, particularly feeding. This brings a harmonious atmosphere into the life of the family, especially if they are also allowed to perform small duties for the new baby.

Family experiences like these help in forming character and they provide the foundation for the development of a responsible attitude towards other human beings later on.

Chapter Three

THE BIRTH

Confinement at home or in hospital?

This question requires careful consideration, for while the hospital may be well equipped to deal with all kinds of emergencies, it also has dangers and disadvantages which are not present in the home. Because there are so many people in a hospital there is a greater danger of infections such as mastitis (inflammation of the breast), influenza, pemphigus of the newborn, and also now epidemic gastro-enteritis, which is the consequence of the indiscriminate use of penicillin and other antibiotics.

The final decision as to where the confinement shall take place is made when the mother is medically examined at the end of the seventh or beginning of the eighth month. The birth will have to be in hospital if the mother's pelvis is too narrow, if a multiple birth is expected, if the child is in an awkward position, or if there are signs of a toxaemia or other illnesses in the mother.

If it is not possible to have the baby at home there are a number of points which must influence the choice of hospital. Above all it must be one where the importance of breast feeding is recognised. In so many places today shortage of staff or insufficiently trained personnel mean that the little perseverance needed to establish the mothers' supply of milk is not forthcoming and the babies are bottle-fed from the beginning on cow's milk and baby foods. The hospital chosen should also be one where the baby's cot remains beside the mother's bed all the time, only being removed at night if the child is very restless. And finally, the mother must make it clear beforehand that she does not wish the vernix to be washed away when the baby is born. This is the slippery substance covering the baby at birth. (See page 64).

The mother's case should be ready packed at least eight weeks before the expected date of birth. It should contain three or more nightdresses which unbutton at the front down to the waist and which can be boiled, a woollen bedjacket, dressing gown, slippers and personal toilet things. Also clothes for the journey home for mother and baby.

For a confinement at home the room where the birth is to take place must be large enough and it is essential that it can be properly heated. Arrangements must be made beforehand to ensure that enough skilled help will be available for mother and baby, so that the baby is not laid aside while the midwife finishes attending to the mother. The midwife or doctor will tell the mother about the various articles she will have to have ready. These will include freshly washed and ironed garments for the child. Ironing is the best way to make laundry sufficiently germ-free.

Painless childbirth

No responsible doctor can promise a woman a completely painless confinement, but it is the duty of the doctor to relieve pain and therefore also the pangs of birth. Dr. Grantly Dick Read's method of natural childbirth (see his books *Natural Childbirth* and *Childbirth without Fear*) can be highly recommended, especially as pain reduction is achieved not by the use of drugs but by the mother's own conscious effort. (Dr. zur Linden would have found the ideas of Professor Leboyer, had he known of them before his death, to be very much in harmony with his own concepts. Ed.)

The beginning of the birth

There are three signs which herald the beginning of the baby's birth: the painless loss of blood and mucous, the painless 'breaking of the waters' which can occur in a sudden flood or just a trickle, and the beginning of labour pains. The latter are caused by contractions of the muscles of the womb and resemble the pains of the monthly period. At first they occur at intervals of twenty to thirty minutes, and when the intervals have decreased to five minutes or less the birth is likely to begin.

Any one of these three signs indicates that the birth is soon to begin, and they can occur in any order. The mother should not wait till all three have manifested. As soon as the first sign occurs she should contact the midwife if the baby is to be born at home, or set in motion the arrangements made for her journey to the hospital.

There is no need for fear or anxiety. The new mother will surely manage what countless women have achieved before her and she can have confidence that what is expected of her will be no more than she can bear.

The birth process

During the first stage of labour the cervix and the rest of the birth canal are rhythmically widened to allow the child to pass through. If the mother relaxes and fearlessly allows this to happen quite automatically, she will experience hardly any pain. But if she interferes in nature's work, the pain will occur. As Dr Read says: 'Tense woman - tense cervix'. Of course the atmosphere in the room and the mother's relationship with the doctor or midwife should be one of confidence and trust.

When the second stage of labour is reached, the time comes for the mother to take an active part in the bearing-down effort, helping to push the child through the birth canal. This activity gives her great satisfaction and she experiences immense joy at being able to help in her baby's birth. With her help the first part of the child, usually the head, emerges from the birth canal. With the next contraction the body will follow and the child is born. The birth process concludes with the emergence of the afterbirth, which consists of the placenta, the amniotic sheaths and the remainder of the umbilical cord.

THE POST-NATAL PERIOD

The first few weeks

Although pregnancy and birth are not illnesses, they do place considerable physical and psychological strain on the mother and she does need time to recover. However long or short her actual time in bed may be (this varies in different countries) she will need a great deal of rest and should sleep whenever she has the opportunity, especially after breast feeding.

Suitable gymnastics, exercises, massage, and also breast feeding all help the womb to return to its normal size and the tummy muscles to regain their usual firmness.

Many mothers sleep badly at first. This is a sign of their inner tension. Recognition of this is in many cases all that is required to help the mother become more relaxed and able to enjoy her baby. Weleda Sedative Tea is also a great help, and often a herbal remedy for stimulating the circulation is the best sleeping draught. Weleda Blackthorn Elixir also helps promote sleep as well as acting as a tonic and stimulating the production of milk. Sleeping tablets should not be taken because the chemical substances they contain are passed on to the baby with the mother's milk.

As a general tonic and also to help prevent thrombosis or inflammation of the veins it is good to take five drops of Arnica D4 with some water three times daily before meals for the first four to six weeks.

Post-natal ailments

After the birth of the baby an open wound is left in the womb which takes a little while to heal. So long as the midwife has been scrupulously clean and done all she should, the mother's own forces of recovery will be sufficient, particularly if she is sensible and has a good quality diet.

Even a cold or mild flu or bronchitis could endanger the mother, and infections like throat inflammations or furunculosis are even more dangerous.

The mother should take her temperature in the morning when she awakes and in the afternoon at about 4 p.m. Taken under the arm it should not exceed 99.5°F (37.5°C). If it rises above 100.4°F (38°C) it could be a sign of incipient mastitis or at least a retention of milk. (It is not certain whether the commencement of lactation causes the temperature to rise as well.) A rise in temperature could also be a sign of trouble in one of the abdominal organs.

Until the wound in the womb has healed entirely, the mother will continue to have a discharge called lochia. This can start to decompose and become rather malodorous. In this case the mother's temperature will rise above 100.4°F (38°C) and she will feel a pressure in the head and general discomfort. The symptoms will be similar if the flow of the lochia becomes congested. Both disturbances can occur during the first eight to ten days after the birth and are easily treated by the doctor who should always be called if there is a rise in temperature.

If the mother's temperature is over 101.3°F (38.5°C) for several days and there are no signs of mastitis or the other ailments mentioned above, she may be found to have infectious childbed fever. If this is so she must be cared for by a private nurse or isolated in hospital so that other women who have just had their babies are not infected. Mother and child may not be nursed by the same person.

Childbed fever usually begins on the third or fourth day after the birth with shivering and a sudden rise in temperature of 104°F (40°C) or more. This could also be a sign of serious mastitis, but whatever is suspected the doctor must be called immediately. Fortunately childbed fever is rare nowadays.

Arnica D4 has already been mentioned as a good tonic and preventative against vein inflammation and embolism. This can be taken from the birth onwards for four to six weeks (5 drops 3 times daily in a little water before meals).

Chapter Five

THE BREAST-FEEDING PERIOD

Diet during breast feeding

Mother's milk is a complete and perfect organism and its value for the child cannot be stressed too highly. Almost without exception breast-fed babies develop harmoniously and without disturbance. Four or five months breast feeding provides a basis for good health throughout life. Even the best substitute cannot provide the resistance to diseases given by mother's milk. In view of all this, surely the mother's great wish must be to provide this blessing for her child, while re-membering that not only her eating habits but also her state of mind, whether she is worried and anxious or calm and loving, affects the child through breast feeding.

The nursing mother's diet should be easily digestible and rich in vitamins and minerals and must include sufficient protein. The quality of the food should be as good as possible. This is because the substances in mother's milk are taken from the food she eats rather more directly than is the nourishment she herself derives from the food. The baby, on the other hand, can only digest normal milk. Thus the mother must expect anything she eats to be reflected quite soon in her milk and then in her baby.

For instance if the mother has taken some wine, she should not be surprised if her baby falls asleep during his next feed instead of drinking his fill. All stimulants which are toxic for adults also damage the baby via the mother's milk. Alcohol and nicotine should therefore be avoided and great care taken with tea and coffee.

Natural and ordinary foods also contain substances which pass over into the milk and some of these might disagree with the baby. For instance cabbage eaten by the mother can cause wind and colic in the baby. Some fruit juices, for example pineapple, strawberry, currant, orange, lemon and tomato, when taken by the mother, can cause nappy rash, nettle rash or other rashes in the baby. Even if she eats honey this can cause diarrhoea in the baby. Careful observation will soon show what foods the mother might have to avoid during the breast feeding period.

Mothers who have to take medicines, especially drugs, must discuss this carefully with their doctor in relation to breast feeding, and in some cases it might be advisable not to breast feed. Special mention may be made of sleeping tablets, tranquillizers, antibiotics, sulphonamides, laxatives, steroids and drugs for asthma, heart and circulation.

If meat is desired, it is best to choose the lean white meat of young animals. But protein requirements should be covered mainly with curd cheese (see recipe page 209), cottage and cream cheese and other mild cheeses that do not smell too strong. Since many nursing mothers as well as their babies suffer from wind, it is useful to add caraway seeds to the water when boiling potatoes and other vegetables or to choose a cheese flavoured with caraway. A cup of caraway seed tea is also a help: Boil a large pinch of the seeds in enough water for a large cup for 10 to 15 minutes.

Bread is often the cause of flatulence, so choose brands baked with caraway or fennel seeds. Demeter bread and Demeter rusks are also recommended.

Main meals should start with 1 to 3 dessertspoons of grated raw vegetables, especially carrots, possibly mixed with a little cream. It is important, however, that these raw vegetables are grown without the use of chemical fertilisers or insecticides.

Raw fruit is also important, and could alternate with the raw vegetables at the start of the main meals. Or else it is eaten between meals.

The evening meal should not be eaten after 6 p.m. or so, since the digestive process slows down over night. Food eaten later remains undigested and weighs on the stomach, pressing on the heart and causing flatulence.

If the mother puts on too much weight, thick soups, puddings and potatoes can be avoided. On the other hand, if she loses weight rapidly she should consult the doctor immediately. It is enough if she weighs herself every two to three weeks.

Beverages will be discussed on page 62.

Menstruation after childbirth

If the mother does not breast feed her baby she will usually have her first period, a rather heavy one, a month after the birth, and after that her periods will be as usual.

Nursing mothers usually remain without a period until they wean the baby. However, about six or eight weeks after the birth it is quite common for nursing mothers to have one rather heavy period. This is quite normal and gives no cause for concern. The baby will be seen to drink his mother's milk with less relish than usual, but there is no need to stop feeding him because of this.

It is quite possible for a woman to become pregnant again while still breast feeding. Three or four weeks after the birth a new egg is released from the ovaries ready for fertilisation. So even if there is no monthly period during breast feeding, a new pregnancy is a possibility.

Six or eight weeks after a normal birth the mother should be examined by a gynaecologist so that he can ascertain whether all her abdominal organs have regained their normal size and position. Once this is found to be so, marital intercourse can be resumed.

The technique of breast feeding

The mother should offer her baby the breast not later than six or eight hours after birth so that he learns to take the nipple and sucks a few times. He will not yet receive much food but this early sucking eases and speeds up the production of milk and when the secretion finally starts it will be less uncomfortable.

During the first few days the mother will feed the baby in bed. She should wash her hands and wipe the nipple with a clean cloth or cotton wool soaked in boiled water. Do not use alcohol or a disinfectant but try to be scrupulously clean without these. The mother lies on her side and relaxes, supported as comfortably as possible by pillows. The baby's nappy is changed and

he is then placed with his head level with the nipple.
Now the mother grasps the areola with the fore and
middle finger of her free hand and presses the nipple
outwards. The outer hand guides the infant's head so
that his mouth touches the nipple. He will instinctively
open his mouth and grasp the nipple and part of the
areola so tightly that when he moves his jaw backwards
a vacuum forms in his mouth into which the milk flows.
The mother should make sure the baby's nose is free for
breathing.

This sucking is quite strenuous. During the course
of a normal period of breast feeding the baby ac-
complishes it about a million times. It promotes a
healthy development of teeth and jaws which is lacking
for the most part if the baby only has a bottle teat to
suck.

Once the mother is up and about she will need a
comfortable chair for feeding, with a footstool high
enough to ensure that the baby lying on her knee on a
pillow can reach the breast without pulling at it. Her
back, arms and legs must be quite relaxed and the baby
must be able to lie in a natural position with the arm he
is lying on quite comfortable. Both mother and baby
must be warm during feeding. The baby can be
wrapped in a light shawl and the mother's arms and
shoulders should be covered. If the room is quiet and
there is nothing to distract him he will concentrate
entirely on drinking.

He will take most of his feed during the first three
minutes, after which it is good to pause. To detach him
the mother may have to hold his nose gently so that he

opens his mouth to breathe. He is held upright so that he can more easily bring up the air he has swallowed. It can be a help to pat him gently on the lower half of his back. After several burps he is put to the breast again and allowed to drink till he is satisfied or falls asleep. The milk is more fatty towards the end of the meal but the amount he drinks is far smaller. If he is allowed to suck too long the nipples get sore and this can lead to an inflammation.

As soon as he stops drinking heartily or starts playing or going to sleep the meal should be finished. He will then be hungrier at the next meal and will soon develop regular habits without being forced. This should, however, not be done unless he is quite healthy.

If the first breast is empty and the child still hungry, there is no harm in giving him the second. This will probably be quite a regular occurrence in the early weeks and it is a good idea to do it anyway at the evening meal. But the mother must ensure that the breast given first is absolutely empty.

At the end of the meal the baby should again bring up as much wind as possible, otherwise it will disturb his digestion and the pain will make him cry.

And finally the mother should rub the nipples with a few drops of lemon juice. She will find a proper nursing brassiere with disposable pads a great advantage.

Emptying the breast
The baby should not be offered the second breast until the first is absolutely drained. If he is persistently unsatisfied after drinking from a particular breast he

should be weighed before and after drinking from that breast to see whether it really contains too little milk.

A breast pump can be used to test whether the first breast is absolutely empty. This is easier but not so effective as milking with the hand, which is best done while seated. The mother takes hold of the breast with both hands, her thumbs uppermost. Stroking the breast with the thumbs from the base towards the nipple she expels the remaining milk. Some women are quite skilled at doing this with only one hand. If there is a lot of milk it can be collected in a sterile container and given to the baby later.

If the first breast is not completely emptied, there is a danger of inflammation with all its undesirable consequences. So the baby must on no account be offered the second breast until the first is empty. If the first breast contains more milk than the baby requires it must likewise be emptied completely with a pump or by milking as described. After each use the pump must be boiled in water with soda and stored in a cloth sterilised by ironing.

The duration of breast feeding

The most normal and desirable timing is to feed a baby entirely on the breast for five months and then to start gradually weaning till he receives no more breast milk at nine months. Even if the mother still has plenty of milk it is not good to breast feed for longer than this, as babies receiving only breast milk after nine months can start suffering from anaemia.

Furthermore the point is missed when the next step

in loosening the ties between mother and child should take place. This step consists in the baby becoming nutritionally independent of the mother. It is the age when he learns to sit and stand. It is time for him to learn to chew and he can start sitting at table with the family. Nutrition is an 'educational aid' and by this change in feeding habits the baby is taught a certain kind of independence.

It is a mistake to assume that continued breast feeding will prevent a new pregnancy.

Weaning

Weaning should be done slowly because too rapid a transition to cow's milk can cause digestive disturbances. This is particularly the case if for some reason weaning has to start before the fifth month. It is usually best to avoid weaning during the hottest weeks of the year.

There is not much the mother need do in order to reduce her milk supply. She can drink less and make sure there is no sign of constipation. If despite this she suffers from retention of milk she should apply lukewarm compresses with Weleda Oak Bark Solution (20%) to the breasts morning and evening and wear a firm brassiere.

During the first week of weaning, one meal is replaced by a bottle feed; the second or third meal is usually the best. In the second week a further feed is replaced by a meal of strained vegetables or rusks (preferably Holle Rusks) soaked in milk. It is possible to proceed like this week by week or to take things more slowly, depending on the child and on the schedule of the baby food chosen to replace the breast (see page 101). Great care must be taken in weaning babies who are not quite well, and if there is acute illness this should be cured before weaning starts.

Inability or refusal to breast feed

There are indeed women who have no milk, but with the majority of those unable to breast feed the reason lies in mistakes during early attempts, mistakes which could be easily avoided.

Unfortunately many maternity hospitals still do not do enough to persuade mothers to breast feed. Often injections given during or after the birth cause insufficient or delayed lactation. Many laxatives and sleeping pills also inhibit lactation directly or else they indirectly affect the child, making him sleepy or giving him diarrhoea so that he does not drink enough. Babies with jaundice of the newborn are also too tired to drink properly.

No doubt there will always be a few women whose vanity prevents them from breast feeding for fear of damage to their figure. This fear is unfounded if the breasts are treated properly during pregnancy and breast feeding. Indeed, breast feeding is positively helpful for the contraction of the abdominal organs. Too little activity and unsuitable brassieres are what make the breast tissues slack. Swimming is a very good regular sport for keeping the tissues firm. Not to breast feed for egoistic reasons is totally irresponsible. It is even thought that women who have milk but do not breast feed are more prone to breast cancer in later years.

There are some rare disturbances which make breast feeding difficult. For instance retracted nipples make it impossible for the baby to take hold and suck. But this condition can for the most part be greatly improved during pregnancy. Several times daily the nipples are sucked out with a breast pump, and wearing nipple shields also helps. In rare cases when they do not improve, the milk can be withdrawn with a breast pump and given to the baby in a bottle. This calls for skill and perseverance but mothers who really know the value of breast milk will gladly undertake the task for several months.

Varying degrees of galactorrhea can occur. In cases where the loss of milk is constant though not great, absorbent pads changed frequently to avoid infection can be used to catch the drips. In serious cases the breast can lose most of its milk.

There are also conditions in which the breasts do not release the milk easily. This is most acute when milk secretion starts very suddenly. It is then necessary to loosen the milk by expelling some either manually or with a breast pump until the breast is less taut.

There are newborn babies who are too weak to suck by themselves, for instance some premature babies. They can be fed on milk obtained from the mother with a breast pump. Indeed, more than any these weak or premature babies need their own mother's milk.

Babies with deformed jaws, for instance a cleft palate, are also unable to suck from the breast and they too can be fed on mother's milk drawn off with a pump. These babies often have a tenacious will to live and they thrive almost without help.

Any noticeable clumsiness in sucking should be pointed out to the paediatrician who should also be consulted if the baby is consistently lazy about drinking.

Sudden shock or excitement can 'make the milk go away'. In fact the milk does not dry up but the ducts are closed by the sudden cramp of shock. In the case of shock the mother should calm down again as quickly as possible, if necessary with the help of 20 drops of valerian tincture in half a glass of sugar water. Any known source of sudden shocks should be avoided, for example television and cinema.

Improving the milk supply

The mother should sleep as much as she can and not do too much physical work if possible. She should drink about two pints (1 litre) over and above what her thirst requires and part of this can consist of three cups daily of Weleda Lactagogue Tea. Apart from its properties of stimulating the milk supply it also has a soothing effect on the digestion of mother and baby and helps combat flatulence in both. However, more than three cups daily can cause diarrhoea in the baby, so the rest of her liquid intake should vary. Milk (butter milk, sour milk and yogurt), herb teas, grain coffee, fruit juices, elixirs are all suitable, but coffee, ordinary tea (except very occasionally), cola drinks and alcohol are not. Smoking is definitely undesirable for the whole period of breast feeding.

Weleda also make a very effective Lactagogue Oil for massaging the breasts several times daily. The resulting increase in the milk supply is often astounding. The oil is warming and greatly stimulates the circulation

Preventing mastitis (inflammation of the breasts)

The mother must always wash her hands thoroughly before feeding and then wash the nipple with plain water. It is good to loosen the milk first by a little gentle massage from the base of the breast towards the nipple. At the end of the feed it is essential to ensure that the breast is absolutely empty before cleaning the nipple with a few drops of lemon juice. The mother must keep her arms warm, specially during feeding.

If a lump appears anywhere in the breast during the feeding period, the breast must be very carefully emptied, if necessary with the help of a breast pump and gentle massage. Then it is lifted firmly with a bandage and if possible the mother should go to bed. If she has a temperature the doctor must be called. Meanwhile a poultice with a thick layer of cool curd cheese is an old remedy for effectively soothing and relieving the pain.

Chapter Six

THE BABY IMMEDIATELY AFTER BIRTH

The newborn baby

At last the time comes when the birth has been happily achieved and the newborn baby lies in his mother's arms. Having heard his first cry and made sure that he is really alive, she now experiences in her soul an entirely new feeling of utter happiness. She may touch him, kiss him, look at him, the most beautiful baby in the world, her very own.

As soon as he arrives the baby begins to adjust to his new surroundings, while the first of so many tasks are performed for him. The umbilical cord is cut and he is quickly rinsed with warm water and then carefully dabbed dry with a warmed towel to ensure that the valuable vernix is not damaged. It should be removed only from face and hands.

This fatty, slippery substance, which entirely covers the baby, first helps him slip through the narrow birth canal. That it then also has other uses is becoming increasingly recognised. Apart from fats it contains mineral salts, vitamins and substances akin to protein. Some midwives know that it protects the skin, for they use it themselves to improve their own complexion. It inhibits the germs with which the baby is surrounded in his new environment, it insulates him and keeps him warm, and finally it is a form of nourishment and is absorbed by his skin within a few days. I have frequently observed that if an infant contracts jaundice of the newborn, which can be rather serious, he has the illness very lightly if he has not had this protective layer removed.

When he is dry he is weighed and measured and then quickly dressed in warmed clothes, placed in his cradle with a hot water bottle (not too hot!) and left in peace to recover from the strains and stresses of being born.

From the moment the umbilical cord is severed changes start taking place within, which are quite difficult for non-medical people to grasp. These changes are particularly prodigious during the first few days of life and one can only assist the infant by keeping him warm and absolutely quiet. The warmth of love with which the parents receive him is not enough on its own. He also needs a great deal of physical warmth particularly in the early weeks.

The severing of the umbilical cord separates the baby physically from his mother. Having received oxygen through his mother's blood he now has to take in with his own lungs the air he will have to share with all of us. He has become our contemporary and fellow citizen.

The baby's first breath brings about a considerable redirection of the blood circulation which before birth by-passed the lungs. Now the wall between the right and the left half of the heart closes and the blood has to circulate through the lungs, refreshing itself there before streaming through the whole body. This very first breath initiates a breaking-down process which is quite prodigious. The embryo has almost twice as many red blood corpuscles as a healthy adult, so within a few hours or days of birth the number of these corpuscles must be halved. Billions of red blood corpuscles perish every minute until the number has decreased from seven or eight million to four million per cubic milli-metre. All these decomposing blood cells have to be dealt with by the digestive organs, particularly the liver. To cope properly the baby needs a great deal of warmth, for of all the organs the liver needs the most warmth. If not kept warm enough the newborn baby might contract serious jaundice which can be dangerous.

An early sign of the breaking-down processes is seen in the activities of the bowel and bladder. First the bowels excrete meconium, a greenish black substance consisting of thickened digestive juices, uterine fluid swallowed by the baby, cells from the walls of the intestines and fine hair from the embryo's skin. This usually takes three or four days and then the baby starts producing the golden-yellow, sweet-smelling motions of a purely milk diet. During the first few days the baby drinks very little milk and therefore passes water only once or twice a day. Later this happens up to thirty times a day. The first urine passed soon after birth is sometimes reddish in colour due to the salts dissolved in it. This is quite harmless.

The rapid smoothing of the baby's wrinkly skin, the adjustment of the skull bones which are often alarmingly squashed, the starting of metabolism in the mouth, the gullet, the stomach and the intestines, all these are wonderful processes which occur soon after birth. But the most wonderful is the gradual regulating of breath and heartbeat till there are about four heartbeats to every breath. From the very first breath the rhythmical activity of heart and lungs begins, never to cease or tire till the last breath. This is one of the great mysteries of life.

At birth the mucous membranes of the air passages and the intestines are completely sterile, but they are soon well provided with beneficial bacteria. A baby sneezes ten or eleven times a day. This helps clear the nose and is not a sign of a cold unless the sneezing is more frequent.

The newborn infant has only reflex reactions to external stimulation of his sense organs and his movements are without any guidance from the brain. This is interesting since it shows that the limbs can indeed move without any help from brain or spinal cord, though such movement is haphazard and aimless.

Some useful figures

A baby is termed newborn until the external signs of the separation of his organism from that of his mother have been overcome, in particular until the remains of the umbilical cord have dropped off. This happens after 8 to 14 days.

At birth, boys are an average 20 to 21 inches (50 to 54cm) long, girls ¾ inch (2cm) less.

Average growth:

in the first month: 1½ to 2 inches (4 to 5cm)

in the second and third months: 1¼ inches (3cm) each

in the fourth and fifth months: ¾ to 1¼ inches (2 to 3cm) each up to the twelfth month: ¼ to ½ inch (1 to 2cm) per month.

At twelve months the average length is 29½ inches (75cm).

At twenty-four months the average length is 33 inches (85cm).

Normal birth weight is anything between 11 lbs (5000g) and 4 lbs 8 oz (2000g), but babies weighing less than 4 lbs 8 oz (2000g) are premature unless it is a case of twins.

After birth babies usually lose between 5 and 10 ozs (150 to 300g) in weight, but the loss is considerably less if the vernix is not removed from the skin. Then from the fourth or sixth day onwards weight is gained again until between the eighth and fifteenth day the birth weight is reached once more. Fairly often this takes considerably longer.

During the first two to three months the daily increase in weight is about ¾ oz (20 to 30g). However, some babies gain up to 1½ ozs (40g) daily and others as little as just over ½ oz (20g). A well-fed baby doubles his birth weight during the fifth month and trebles it during the eleventh or twelfth month. At the end of the second year his weight will have quadrupled. If the weight at birth was relatively low, the increase will be more rapid.

Breast-fed babies and those fed on Holle Baby Food gain weight evenly, while babies fed on other baby mixtures tend to gain in fits and starts. It is quite easy to increase a baby's weight considerably. But the real art of nutrition lies in avoiding any over-feeding. In cases of illness, overweight children are in greater danger than those with the correct weight.

First examination by the doctor

If possible the baby should be examined by the doctor on the first day of his life. For me this is still as happy and exciting a task as it was forty years ago.

First I look at the general appearance of this new little boy or girl. Is the skin smooth and pink or wrinkled and shrivelled like that of an old person? From this I can tell whether the birth was lengthy or fairly quick, whether it was late or at the right time, and whether the infant will soon need some milk or can wait a while longer. On the first or second day the skin should not yet show any yellowness. At the back of the head or neck and near the eyes many newborn babies have harmless birthmarks which later vanish.

I examine the fine hair which often covers the whole body; I look at the lines in the palms of the hands and on the soles of the feet and at the length of the finger and toe nails. I examine the shape of the whole body and compare the size of the head with that of the chest. Length and weight are the most important measurements for determining the maturity of the newborn. A baby who is too short, underweight, very hairy, has only feeble reactions to external stimuli, i.e. touch and temperature, and one who lacks the sucking reflex is likely to be immature.

Then I examine the head to see whether there are any swellings or whether the bones of the skull, which are still very mobile, are pressed together. I feel the fontanels and the seams between the bones with my fingers. They are not yet fixed or closed, so they can give way to pressure during birth, to any fluctuations of blood pressure in the head, and also accommodate the rapid growth of the brain. The large fontanel is at the top of the head and is the spot where the brain is only protected by some tough skins. Through these one can feel the blood pulsating in the head. The small fontanel is at the back of the head.

The significance of the fontanels is probably much greater than we have realised hitherto. The small one closes soon after birth, but the large fontanel should not be entirely closed until the child is eighteen months old. Nowadays certain diets and excessive prescriptions of vitamin D cause the fontanel to close too soon, as early as ten months sometimes. (See page 138ff and 142ff).

Then with the help of a spatula or small spoon I examine the cavity of the mouth and palate. Various malformations are possible here which an operation later on can correct, but which meanwhile could cause the child difficulty in sucking.

After this I make sure there is no wry-neck, where the head is drawn to one side by shortened neck muscles. I feel the spine from top to bottom and make sure that all the joints and muscles of the arms and legs work properly and that there are the correct number of fingers and toes.

The state of the navel is examined very carefully. I show the mother how to treat it properly with a sterile dressing fixed in position by a bandage wound round the baby's body starting from below the navel and working upwards, like laying tiles on a roof, to ensure that it will not slip.

Then I listen to the heart with my stethoscope in case there is any congenital abnormality. Normally a newborn baby has one hundred and forty heartbeats and about fifty-five breaths a minute. But frequently soon after birth the heart and lung rhythms have not yet adjusted themselves. The doctor must then make regular examinations until the adjustment is made, which is usually after about six weeks.

Now the abdomen is examined. I feel the liver, which is normally large at this age, and the size of the spleen is noted. The firmness of the abdominal walls is felt in case there are any weak spots where ruptures might occur. The genitals and the anus are examined.

Finally I look at the visible part of the baby's ears, their shape, size, proportions, angle to the head, the differences between right and left and whether they are delicate or coarse. The external ear reveals a great deal about the physical and soul characteristics of the new human being. Heredity alone cannot explain the infinite variety in the shape of people's ears.

The mother's nerves

A mother with a new baby, especially if it is her first, tends to be far too worried and cramped. In trying to do everything perfectly she easily overreaches herself, becoming more and more ill at ease and losing her inner balance. Fears for the child's health and even his life keep her awake at night; and every time he cries her nerves become more strained. At the same time during the puerperal period of six to eight weeks she herself is only gradually recuperating from the strain of the baby's birth.

Usually the mother copes with all this unaccustomed strain for six or seven weeks, but then her nerves give way and she dissolves into tears and despair. She thinks she will never be a capable mother or have enough strength to master her new tasks properly.

However, if she knows there is likely to be this crisis after six or seven weeks she can take precautions in time. Perhaps she has a mother or sister who can help her in the house. She can take more rest, go for regular walks and drink a soothing tea before going to bed (e.g. Weleda Sedative Tea). But above all she must try and become more relaxed in her attitude towards the baby. He will thrive the better if she is at ease and calm.

If she knows these things the new mother will soon be able to laugh at her tears and overcome the crisis in a few days. She should know, however, that when the baby is about three months old there may be another similar crisis and a further one sometimes occurs at nine months.

Peace and quiet and the quality of care
The baby is totally unable to protect himself from his surroundings so it is up to the adults around him, particularly his mother, to select for him the impressions which can help him. During the very early weeks he should be kept really quiet, but soon there are many noises which can go on around him without being harmful. Ordinary household work and the sound of

older brothers and sisters at play and people talking are noises to which he should soon become accustomed and which are in no way harmful. But he should be protected from mechanical noise, even that of the vacuum cleaner, for as long as possible. Sounds from radio and television are totally alien for him. Music that reaches his ears indirectly via electrically generated waves is quite unsuitable, whereas live music, especially singing and lyre playing, is helpful for the child.

Not only physical noise and bustle or garish lights or cold but also emotional disturbances, anger, quarrelling or hatred have direct effects on the child's development.

Adherence to a strict daily rhythm, both in feeding and general care, greatly helps the baby to establish the regular functioning of all his organs.

The mother should try not to be too anxious about the child, for unless she makes a really bad mistake she is not likely to do him much harm. Sensible caution is quite different from anxiety. Besides, raising a child requires a certain degree of faith in God in addition to reliance on one's own intelligence. Two valuable hints can help the mother decide for herself whether the baby is in danger. Firstly, though there are some exceptions, a healthy baby's arms usually lie on the pillow on either side of his head, when he sleeps, rather than down by his sides. Think of a healthy plant with its leaves raised up or a wilting plant with its leaves drooping. Secondly the mother should pay attention to the delicate fragrance which emanates from her baby. If he is well, this fragrance will remain until he begins to teethe at about nine months when he also starts to eat solid food. If it disappears earlier it is a sign that the baby is ailing, for instance there might be incipient rickets.

After only a few days or weeks the mother will know from the way her baby is crying whether he is thirsty, or whether the trouble is tummy ache or wet nappies. It will also not be long before she can distinguish the crying of her own baby from that of others.

The uniqueness of the baby's cry is one of the first tentative signs of this child's individual human qualities.

The average rate of development

The age at which children learn each new skill is not fixed, so the following timing is only an approximate guide.

First the newborn baby develops all the functions needed for preserving life. Thus nearly every infant learns very quickly how to take the mother's breast and if the child seems in any way clumsy about this the doctor should be consulted immediately. A few hours after birth babies can suck their fingers loudly. Every infant has his own method, beginning even in this activity to show his individuality.

Babies can taste soon after birth and as mother's milk is sweetish their taste is adjusted to sweet things. A bottle-fed baby soon learns to reject a feed which is not sweet enough. The sense of touch develops early, so that babies begin to notice the discomfort of a fold in the nappy or a change of temperature. Soon after birth they can also hear and they jump at sudden noises. Infants only a few days old can react to colours. In the third week the eyes begin to work together, though they do not yet see properly. The pupils contract when light shines on them. But the baby as yet takes no notice of what is going on round him, sleeping most of the time except when feeding.

From the beginning the baby's facial muscles are amazingly mobile and his grimaces endless. The limbs, too, are very mobile, but the muscles are at first in a state of considerable tension, particularly if the child is chilled. In some babies the head is bent rather far back as a result of the position in the womb. The infant can yawn soon after birth and also sneeze, which he does ten or eleven times a day.

In the second month the baby will start to grasp objects if they touch the palm of his hand. At about six weeks he can lift his head when placed on his stomach. He begins to make small noises and babbles gaily, particularly after meals. Sometimes he will follow a close moving object with his eyes and even turn his head. His first smile appears and also his first tears: the newborn infant's crying is tearless.

In the third month he can turn his head when he hears a noise. His eyes can follow light moving objects. And he recognises things he sees often, such as his mother's face which he greets with a smile.

In the fourth and fifth month he begins to grasp purposefully. He lifts his little arm and practises moving first the hand and then the individual fingers, observing this with his eyes. When taken out of his cot he holds his head up and turns it himself, and he sits upright on his mother's arm. While his nappies are being changed he kicks joyfully. He can turn on to his back from his side or even his tummy. When on his tummy he props himself on his arms. He obviously enjoys all his movements.

During the sixth month he learns to place his feet on the floor and straighten his knees as a preliminary to standing. He can sit up alone and thus discovers more and more about his surroundings, recognising familiar people. He already begins to copy sounds such as clucking noises made with the tongue for his benefit. The room is filled with his joyful chuckling which expresses his good humour and enjoyment of life.

From the seventh to the ninth month all that he has learned so far is perfected. He sits by himself with a straight back on a cushion. He stands holding on to the bars of his playpen and gradually learns to pull himself up on his own. He rolls around his playpen in order to reach his toys. He hardly ceases producing sounds with his mouth, till one day 'mama' or 'dada' is heard for the first time. Fathers of course take it as personal homage if 'dada' is heard first. Whether they are right or not is hard to tell. There are little girls who from the cradle are fascinated by daddy and later by all men! Then the child begins to understand other words, beaming with pleasure for instance when he hears the word 'bottle'. By nine months he should have learnt to chew bread.

Between ten and twelve months he learns to walk to someone calling him if there are enough things to hold on to on the way. He will, however, start being selective, showing sympathy and antipathy clearly towards those around him.

As the child stands and begins to walk at the end of the first year, he now requires freedom to use his limbs and practise as much as possible. Only at night he should be prevented from tumbling about in his bed and ending up completely uncovered.

He eats bread by himself and should begin to drink out of a mug. He should not be allowed to taste any titbits such as cheese or sausage, for this will spoil his taste for his less interesting baby food. He will crawl on all fours, pull himself up on the furniture and walk holding on to it. If led by the hand he will take proper steps. He copies words and sometimes uses them correctly. Children who have been drilled too much will already connect a specific meaning to a word. An eleven and a half month old baby once pointed beaming at the hair on the back of my hand and said 'doggy'.

At eighteen months a child has a vocabulary of about forty words. He should be able to walk and be quite clean and dry during the daytime. Training for this should not start too early. Even nine months is un-necessarily soon, and lengthy potty-sitting often leads to cystitis or other ailments caused by chills.

At two and a half the child can be clean and dry both day and night. This is the time when he also begins for the first time to notice himself as an individual. He no longer feels himself to be a part of his environment but finds that he is a separate person within this environment. Instead of calling himself 'Johnny' he now begins to say 'I', 'I want to have...', 'I want to do...;.

Chapter Seven

CARING FOR THE BABY

The baby's bed

Remembering how protected the baby is in the mother's womb it is obvious that a cot with bars cannot be a very snug place for him once he is born. It is always draughty, however well he is covered. The best bed for the first few weeks is a wickerwork cradle lined with plain pale red or white material. Dots or other patterns are not so suitable. Even a large washing basket will do. This will protect him from draughts and is even a little similar to the womb in shape. The baby needs as much warmth as possible and also protection from all the impressions assailing him in his new surroundings. Therefore a canopy is also necessary. This is best made with pale red silk covered with pale blue silk. Sunlight shining through this makes a wonderfully calming purple glow. Undyed natural silk can also be used. Though blue is a calming colour for adults, small babies are calmed by a beautiful glowing red or better still purple. Light red silk also protects the baby from the inflammatory rays of the sun while letting through those which help prevent rickets. So with the protection of the canopy the baby can be allowed much more sunlight than would otherwise be possible

The mattress should be completely flat, fairly hard and without springs. The best fillings are horsehair or kapok; eelgrass is also quite good. In the olden days mattress stuffing was often of chaff, particularly millet chaff, a warmer and healthier base than many modern mattresses.

A pillow is superfluous but if one is used it should be very thin and of horsehair. This is essential to prevent spinal distortions. Feathers are out of the question because they make the head dangerously hot.

A rubber sheet may be used to protect the mattress but it must be covered with a flannel sheet. Good woollen blankets are the best covering. Cotton is not warm enough and continental quilts are usually too hot and can even be dangerous in hot weather. The blankets can be enclosed in a washable slip with strong tapes at all four corners so that it can be secured under the mattress to ensure that the baby remains covered. When he is older he can be put in a sleeping bag which is also attachable to the four corners of the bed (see page 93).

Rocking the baby

In contrast to most authors on child care I have for many years now been in favour of rocking babies in a cradle.

There is no question of spoiling the child, for only a few minutes of rocking are needed to send him to sleep. The right speed can be found with the help of a lullaby. The rhythmic to and fro resembles breathing in and out and the repeated slight jolt between every swing helps detach the consciousness from the nervous system and send the baby to sleep. The baby can be rocked approximately until he has cut his first teeth, and then he will be ready for an ordinary cot.

It is quite easy to turn a carry cot or basket into a cradle by placing it on a rocking base like that of a rocking horse.

Crying

On the whole a healthy baby with a full tummy and not too wet a nappy does not cry without reason. But some are more restless and cry more readily, for instance if there is a fold in the nappy or if they are bored. These stop as soon as they are attended to. Rudolf Steiner once suggested that a canopy of orange silk might be a help with such children.

At the end of the first month or during the second month, however, there is a period which can last up to four weeks when nearly every baby cries regularly every day for an hour or two and cannot be comforted. So if there is nothing obviously wrong and if the crying takes place at the same time each day, usually towards evening, there is nothing for it but to grit one's teeth and comfort oneself with the knowledge that this is really the baby's first sporting activity which strengthens heart and lungs.

If a baby cries several times a day he usually either has not had enough to drink, which can be difficult to determine with breast-fed babies, or he has a pain, perhaps caused by wind. A little fennel tea will usually comfort him. Boil 1 level teaspoon of fennel seeds in 1 cup of water for 1-3 minutes. Add a little sugar to taste. Some aniseed can be boiled with the fennel if wind is the trouble. Also his mother can pick him up and carry him a little with his head face down in the crook of her arm and her warm hand supporting his tummy while she gently pats his behind with the other hand. Then if she has a cradle she can rock the baby for a few minutes or if not then rock him in her arms.

Weak babies or the babies of older parents are sometimes too quiet and do not cry even if they are hungry.

Nearly all babies cry after feeding until they have brought up swallowed wind (see page 57).

Keeping the baby's abdomen warm

On the whole babies are not kept warm enough nowadays. Except on the hottest days it is hardly possible to keep a baby too warm during the early months.

It is particularly the abdomen which must be kept warm at all times. Chills caught in that region during nappy changing are the most frequent cause for discomfort, pains and hiccups (see page 82).

The damp warmth inside the nappy usually has a temperature of about 98.6°F (37°C) while room temperature is often not more than 65° to 68°F (18° to 20°C). The evaporation caused by this drop of thirty or more degrees F (nineteen C) is a great shock to the system and often results in colic pains or bladder chills and worse. Spring and autumn are the most difficult seasons.

So the room should be as warm as possible when the baby is to be changed. In addition, when the nappy is partly undone it is a good idea to dry underneath it with a towel before opening it completely. Keep the abdomen covered all the time, use warm water and work quickly. The clean nappies should be warmed.

The best way is to keep the next lot of nappies and a change of clothes with the baby in his cot.

Hiccups

A baby who often suffers from lengthy bouts of hiccups, a cramp of the diaphragm, is being treated wrongly in some way. Either his abdomen has been chilled during nappy changing (see above), or his bottle has not been warm enough. When feeding with the bottle it is important to keep it warm with a woollen cover or to warm it up every few minutes in hot water.

The ancient Greek doctor Hippocrates recommended tickling in the nose with a feather as a cure for hiccups. Sneezing stretches the diaphragm and this brings the hiccups to an end. A warm camomile bag laid on the tummy usually does the trick too. Fill a small muslin bag with camomile flowers and heat on the lid of a boiling saucepan. Then place on the baby's tummy.

The dummy

Babies who do not want to suck a great deal should use their fingers. But if a good deal of sucking is done a suitable dummy should be provided because the danger of deforming the gums is too great. This is not only ugly but can affect health. Enormous numbers of children have to undergo corrective treatment after spoiling their gums or teeth by sucking fingers or thumbs. The best dummy is one which causes the baby or small child to suck as it would at the mother's breast. 'NUK Sauger' dummies made in Western Germany are excellent if obtainable.

While teething a baby can wear a necklace of amber beads on which he can bite. A single piece of amber on a ribbon or a ring of ivory or horn, but not plastic, is also good, as is the traditional orrisroot. Dummy sucking should cease latest at the change of teeth.

Should the baby lie mostly on his tummy?

This is frequently recommended, but the reasons given are unconvincing. They seem to stem more than anything from the general tendency to equate human beings with animals. Because dogs and cats lie on their bellies does not mean that this is the best or most 'natural' position for human babies. Indeed, it is more in keeping with the dignity of man not to lie facing the earth, and down the centuries babies have thrived quite happily lying on their backs facing the universe or lying on one or other side. Similarly, the baby is the only creature on earth who can look into his mother's face when being fed. Fortunately, science is at last coming to realise that right from the moment of conception the human being is human and not animal.

Sun bathing

Essential though the rays of the sun are for the baby, it can be very harmful to expose him to them too early or too directly, but there are of course seasons and places with little sunshine which make it necessary to be more generous. The skin should be allowed to tan only slowly. From three or four months onwards in good weather the sun can be allowed to shine on the naked baby's back and tummy for a few minutes, but the head must always be protected. It has been discovered that blue sky is just as effective as direct sunlight.

Daily fresh air

As with everything, a happy medium must be found here. Any attempt to toughen the child can lead merely to a hardening and a dulling of the senses when the aim is to maintain a healthy sensitivity to external stimuli provided for instance by sun, air, water and food. So there should be no enforced exposure, for instance to cold wind.

After the sixth week the baby should have some fresh air daily. At first his cot can be placed by the open window and then when the weather is good his pram can be left for many hours on the balcony or in the veranda or garden so long as his head is protected from wind and sun. This is much better than taking him for a walk in the pram. In town the latter should be avoided as long as possible. The noise of cars rushing past shocks the baby and the worst exhaust fumes lie low on the road at the level of many prams. There is much to be said for prams on high wheels so long as the baby is firmly strapped in once he can sit up.

It is equally pointless to take him for a walk in a pram which is completely sealed against the elements. One might as well spare him the jolting.

Babies cool very quickly in a cold wind, so in windy weather their time out of doors must be corresponding-ly shorter. East winds and cold below 21°F (minus 4°C) call for particular caution, extra clothes and coverings, and even a hot water bottle.

Infant gymnastics

Anyone who has observed attentively how babies practise with their little fists, how they watch intently as the fingers open and close and the hand turns in every direction, knows that this is one of the most touching and intimate manifestations of the coming together of body and soul.

And anyone who has also seen an infant gymnast at work, bending and stretching the little limbs backwards and forwards like parts of a machine in a tempo and rhythm quite foreign to the child must realise that this is utter madness and even a crime against the child.

To justify this sort of thing by saying that the babies enjoy it is a dangerous conclusion. Within a few days the infant's healthy instincts can be ruined. Gymnastics at this age start a development which is just as 'good' as the blossoming of a plant in a hot-house. The damage shows years later in weaknesses of the motor system which has been stimulated too early and too unnaturally.

It is quite another matter if the mother gently and playfully stimulates the baby to use his limbs. She can let him push against her hand with his feet or she can place him on his tummy and encourage him to turn his head. This kind of gentle activity can never be harmful.

Care of skin and hair

The newborn baby's skin is red and usually very sensitive and easily inflamed, particularly during the early weeks.

Except for the first quick rinse after birth the baby

should not be bathed until the navel is completely healed and dry. Washing with lukewarm water and a little baby soap is quite sufficient. The soaps, creams, oils and powders used for the baby should be the purest obtainable and perfumed only by natural ingredients. A special flannel and separate water should be used for the face. If the baby has hair this need not be washed daily. Cotton wool or soft tissues are best for cleaning eyes, nose and ears.

Around the large fontanel babies with hair often have a fatty secretion which takes the form of a greyish scaling. This is quite harmless and without endangering the fontanel it can be softened with oil and then gently scraped off with a comb or a card.

The protective coating of oil in the baby's skin can be enhanced with the application of a pure vegetable oil once a week, any surplus being removed with a towel. This is particularly beneficial for weak babies who feel the cold easily. Weleda Hypericum Oil is very good.

Those parts of the skin which are constantly in contact with wet and dirty nappies may need protecting with oil or cream.

The baby's hair can be brushed with a soft brush with natural bristles. A brush which is too hard stimulates the secretion of oil. It is unlikely that brushing or combing might damage the fontanel.

Nappies

Since a baby wets his nappy up to thirty times a day it is impossible to change him every time. He should be changed before every meal and once or twice in between if he cries to show that he is uncomfortable. This applies to the night as well, but one or at the most two changes will do at night if he does not cry. Most babies produce a dirty nappy up to three times a day and when this happens they should be changed immediately. Usually mothers will find themselves changing nappies about seven times a day at first. They should be able to accomplish this very quickly and without disturbing the baby.

Whatever nappies are used, the final result of the nappy procedure should be a firm bundle, especially in the first three months. A shawl wrapped neatly round everything else is a good way of achieving this. If possible wait till the baby is older before using disposable nappies.

Plastic pants are very undesirable. They cause overheating of the abdomen which leads to an even greater risk of chill when the nappies are changed. They also probably cause certain components of the urine to be absorbed by the skin. Many babies get sore when plastic pants are used. If it is impossible to manage without, a plastic square which does not make the nappy bundle airtight can be used.

Bathing

Daily bathing is undesirable, especially when it means the daily use of soap. The baby's bottom is washed several times a day anyway and the rest of him is not likely to get too dirty. Apart from the fact that bathing is very strenuous for many babies, soap deprives the skin of the valuable oils which help keep him warm and protect him from infection and various external irritations. It cannot be replaced by even the finest oil applied externally. When oil is used on the baby's skin it should be vegetable oil and definitely not mineral or tar based.

Bathing should always take place before a meal, never after. In winter twice and in summer three times a week is quite sufficient. After the first few months well covered babies can be bathed more often. The temperature of the water should be 97°F (36°C) and the room at least 68°F (20°C). Soon the mother will learn to use her elbow to ascertain the correct water temperature. The baby should not be in the water for more than five minutes. Since windows and doors should remain closed, everything must be prepared in advance and placed within reach of the mother's free hand: water thermometer, bowl of lukewarm water for the face, flannel for the face, flannel for the rest, cotton wool, container for used cotton wool, baby soap, baby powder, baby cream, oil, towel, clean clothes, hair brush and comb.

Start with the face (do not submerge the ears) and finish with the bottom. With girls sponge from the front backwards between the legs to prevent bacteria from entering the vagina. After the bath dry the baby very carefully all over, in all the folds and the palms of the hands. With girls part the lips of the vagina and wipe carefully from front to back with cotton wool soaked in oil. Powder lightly in all folds, under arms and between legs.

Sleep

The baby's sleep should be regarded as sacrosanct. Never wake him if at all possible, but if once in a while it is necessary then do so very gently. Some babies look very pale while asleep.

During the early weeks babies sleep nearly all day except while being fed and changed. Only hunger, thirst and the discomfort of dirty nappies wake them and they often fall asleep before they have finished a meal.

The regular crying time described earlier (see page 80) falls in the second month, but otherwise the baby still sleeps nearly all the time.

During the third month the baby lies awake for some of the time playing with his hands, kicking with his legs and practising his first sounds. This continues, but by the sixth month he should still be sleeping for twelve to fourteen hours at night and for two or more hours morning and afternoon.

At one year and more he should still sleep twelve hours at night and also some time morning and afternoon.

Every hour of sleep is useful for the child and his development. It should be possible to do ordinary housework and even put on the light without disturbing a good sleeper. Overfed babies and nervously excitable babies usually sleep less than they should.

Swallowing air

If the baby cries for a long time and seems to be in pain, check whether his tummy is swollen and hard

with wind. Babies often swallow air with their food and
this stretches the stomach, pushing up the diaphragm.
This interferes considerably with breathing and the
functioning of the heart and can be most painful. If the
baby has to breathe through his mouth because his nose
is blocked with a cold he is more likely to swallow air
while feeding. Quite often a drink of just over an ounce
(30g) of caraway seed tea will help. (Boil a large pinch
of caraway seeds in enough water for a large cup for 15
minutes). This diminishes the effect of the wind but it
may not help sufficiently. The doctor may have to
release it by inserting a thin tube into the baby's
stomach. About an ounce (30g) of fennel or aniseed tea
(see page 80) helps with very young babies, combined
with a camomile compress round the abdomen. (see
page 196).

Colds

If the baby has a cold and a blocked nose he will keep
trying to suck and then let go to breathe till he gives up,
crying with frustration. His nose can be cleared with a
weak solution of salt in water inserted into the nostrils
on a blob of cotton wool. Dissolve just over ¼ oz. (9g) of
salt in two pints (1 litre) boiled water. If necessary
follow this with a little Weleda Catarrh Cream inside
and outside the nose.

No one with a cold or flu should be allowed near a
small baby. If the mother herself has a cold she should
wash her hands very carefully before attending to him
and if possible cover her mouth and nose with a mask or
muslin nappy.

Bowel movements

During the first five or six days the bowel excretes meconium, a greenish black substance. After a few days its place is taken by the golden-yellow pleasantly fragrant motions of a purely milk diet. At first there may be up to six motions a day, some of which may be rather liquid or bitty. The motions of a bottle-fed baby are usually greyish yellow in colour, rather firm and stale smelling. After the first week, the baby does not usually pass more than one to two motions in twenty-four hours.

With breast-fed babies, there is no cause for worry if several days pass without a motion, so long as the baby has no tummy pain. The cause may be an insufficient intake of milk, so it is sensible to weigh the baby before and after meals to check the amount he is taking.

Clothes for the baby and small child

As adults we know how uncomfortable it is to feel cold and how it prevents us from working properly either physically or mentally. A baby feels even more uncomfortable and yet he cannot complain. If his mother is observant she will notice what is the matter if he is too pale or if there are disturbances in his development. The soul and spirit need sufficient warmth for their work of moulding and remoulding the body. What is said in this section applies particularly to the first three years.

As far as possible all the baby's clothes should be made of natural materials such as wool, cotton and silk. Synthetic fibres are a very poor substitute.

The baby's vests should be of wool or pure silk. Cotton and linen are not warm enough, particularly for delicate babies without enough fat. A thin woollen vest is the baby's most important item of clothing. So long as it is clean it should be kept on at night.

All fresh clothes should be warmed before they are put on, particularly in winter. A good way is to keep them in the cot with the baby as mentioned above. Otherwise every change of clothing brings about a considerable loss of heat.

However, it must be emphasised that on hot summer days there can be a danger of overheating which can lead to serious diarrhoea. Signs of this are restlessness, a red face and sweaty hair. Therefore let it be said once again that woollen blankets should be used since they allow for ventilation, whereas quilts can retain too much heat (see page 79).

While the baby is wrapped in a fairly firm bundle for the first three months (see section on nappies), at about four months he can start wearing rompers or leggings and is allowed to kick for a few hours each day. But at night he should still be wrapped fairly firmly, though of course never so tightly that he cannot move his legs at all. It seems that the baby needs a fairly firm wrapping until the development of his internal organs has reached a certain stage. This does not mean that he should not be allowed to kick while he is being changed or bathed. As with everything one must find the golden mean. Experience has shown that if the limbs are left too free too early there is a tendency later for scatter-brained lack of concentration, while if they are swaddled too tightly there is a tendency for physical and mental inhibition and clumsiness. As has been said, the soul and spirit work right inside the body and are affected by what they experience in the limbs at this early age.

Towards the end of the first year, when the baby begins to stand, it is time to give his limbs all the freedom they want so that he can learn to use them. But at night he should still be prevented from tossing and turning too much. The continental idea of a warm sack for the body and legs attached to a bodice which leaves the arms free is a very good solution. Tapes attached to the bottom of the sack and to the bodice are fixed under the mattress tightly enough to prevent the child from standing up but slack enough to allow him to turn over. In this way he cannot kick off his bedclothes and catch a chill. The sack has a zip down one side to allow for nappy changing.

When the baby starts to crawl the clothes must be designed to prevent him from catching a chill in the lower part of the body. Heat rises, so the floor is the coldest and draughtiest part of most rooms. Small girls in particular often contract an inflammation of the bladder or worse while they are learning to crawl. They should wear woolly pants, tights and trousers.

The general rule is that the lower part of the body must always be kept warm while the upper part can be exposed much more to the fresh air. The kitchen of the body where the cooking (digestion) takes place is the tummy. To do its work the liver, the most important digestive organ, needs the considerable heat of 102.2° to

105.8°F (39° to 41°C). The child does not have enough strength to create this warmth if its abdomen is not sufficiently clothed. The mother need then not be surprised if he has no appetite, is pale and does not develop properly.

If children wear ankle socks or knee socks their knees and thighs will be far too cold and the chill creeping up towards the abdomen affects not only the work of bladder and liver but also interferes with the development of all the abdominal organs. The consequences in later life are far more serious than most mothers imagine.

A child's foot usually looks completely flat until the third or fourth year because the arch is filled with a cushion of fat which remains until the muscles of the foot are strong enough to carry the weight of the child. The development of the muscles is hindered if the child wears boots or shoes with special supports or soles. So buy good shoes with flexible soles or good sandals. And avoid the X-ray apparatus still used in some shops. They damage the cells in the growing foot, though the consequences do not appear for many years.

Dangers due to carelessness
- Anything pointed is dangerous. Safety pins should only be used if they are so large that even the strongest baby cannot open them.
- Toys with wooden balls or beads should only be given if the balls and beads are too big to be put in the mouth. Mind that older children do not give the baby conkers or marbles!

First aid if something is swallowed: Place the baby on his tummy, support his head and hold his nose so that he opens his mouth. Pat sharply with the flat of the hand on the upper part of the back. If something sharp or spiky is swallowed, feed the baby immediately with semolina pudding or mashed potato and call the doctor!

If an object is blocking the windpipe (the child turns blue!), place a hand on either side of the chest and press sharply. The expelled air will remove the object.

- Care should be taken with bedding. A child can smother himself with a feather pillow. After the third month a baby is safest in a sleeping bag as described on page 93

- Plastic bags are a menace. Children can pull them over mouth and nose and suffocate.

- Babies have been known to strangle themselves with the ribbon to which their dummy is attached. Any ribbons or cords (e.g. on toys or curtains) near the baby are dangerous.

- Babies should not be given any breakable toys, particularly those ugly plastic animals, dolls or rattles.

- All toys must be washable and the paint non-poisonous.

- Babies should not be left alone with animals. It happens again and again that cats sit on babies and smother them. Dogs must not be allowed to lick the baby.

- People with colds or flu should not be allowed near the baby. If the mother has a cold she can tie a nappy round mouth and nose while attending to him. She should also wash her hands thoroughly.

- Babies and children should never travel in the front seat of a car. In an accident they are far safer on the back seat.

Chapter Eight

FEEDING THE BABY

1. BREAST FEEDING

Feeding schedule

Until there is enough milk, which can take up to six weeks, the baby will need six meals a day. The traditional times are 6 a.m., 10 a.m., 2 p.m., 6 p.m., 10 p.m., 2 a.m. This regular sucking every four hours helps to stimulate the supply of milk. Soon the baby will sleep through the night and the 2 a.m. feed can be omitted.

The four-hour gaps between feeds should be maintained as strictly as possible. It is quite all right to wake the baby gently when the next feed is due. His stomach needs just that time to digest the previous meal and rest. While it is right to be regular about the timing of meals it is nonsense to expect the baby to drink exactly the same amount each time and it is quite unnecessary to weigh a healthy baby after every meal.

On the first day the baby can be put to the breast twice but will obtain only a few drops. If the birth was lengthy and the baby is rather dried out with a very wrinkly skin, he can be given a few drops of fennel or camomile tea with a pipette or tiny spoon but he will probably take less than 1/3oz. (10g). The tea can be slightly sweetened.

Proper feeding begins on the second day. The baby is put to the breast six times, though very placid babies who were heavy at birth are usually satisfied with five meals from the start. Given six meals, the amount required will be 1/3 to 2/3oz. (10 to 20g) and given five meals up to 1 oz or just over (30g). During these early days the baby obtains only the colostrum, a thick yellow liquid, so if there is not enough he can be given a little camomile or fennel tea with a spoon. The colostrum is extremely valuable for the baby and he should have every available drop.

On the third day the amount needed will be six times nearly 1 oz (25g) or five times just over an ounce (30g).

And on the fourth day the amount is increased by under 1/4oz. (5g) per meal. By the fifth and sixth day the milk supply starts to be properly established and the baby will need six times about 1¾ oz. (50g) or five times just over 2 oz. (60g).

From the seventh day the amount will increase by about 10g per meal each day. But there are no exact rules and every baby has his own individual needs.

The following rule of thumb may be helpful for calculating the amounts needed in the early weeks.

Up to and including the sixth week the amount of breast milk taken daily should be about one sixth of the baby's weight. For example if the baby weighs 8 lbs (3,600g), the daily amount would be 8 (3,600) ÷ 6 = 21oz approx (600g) or 4¼oz. (120g) for each of five feeds. From the seventh week onwards the baby should take one seventh of his weight. For example if he weighs 10¾ lbs (4,900g) the daily amount would be 10¾ (4,900) ÷ 7 = 1½ lbs (700g), i.e. 5 oz. (140g) for each of five feeds.

Some babies are exceptionally large and they do need

more. However, if given a few teaspoons of un-
sweetened fennel tea before each meal they will drink
less greedily and not exceed the normal amount so
easily.

Some breast-fed babies begin to sleep through the
10 p.m. feed at four or five months and take more in the
morning instead. The daily intake of these babies is
then somewhat less than it would be with five meals,
though they then usually drink more than 7 oz. (200g)
at each feed.

To check the amount taken at a particular feed,
weigh the baby with all his clothes before and after
feeding; and add up the total for the daily intake. If he is
not getting enough, do not immediately try to supplement the breast with cows' milk. Instead try to satisfy
him with a little herb tea or diluted fruit juice. He will
then be hungrier for the next meal and will suck harder,
thus increasing the milk supply.

During the early weeks there is no reason why the
baby should not be given a little drink during the night
if he is thirsty. Give him only a small amount of sweetened herb tea and he will soon get into the habit of
sleeping through the night, since it will not be 'worth his
while' to make a big fuss for nothing but a little tea. If he
does not fall asleep again after he has been changed and
given 2/3 to 1 oz. (20-25g) of herb tea, it may be
presumed that he is not receiving sufficient nourishment during the day, so he must be given more at the
10 p.m. feed or for each feed during the day.

A sixth daily feed is necessary for delicate babies who
cannot take too much food at once and also for strong,

hungry babies. There is no need to let hungry babies cry for hours at night, and after a short time, four to six weeks, the babies will sleep through the night of their own accord. If the baby does wake at night it is essential to change his wet or dirty nappies.

Latest in the eighth week even completely breast-fed babies should begin to have additional foods. A start can be made with a few teaspoons of carrot juice or small amounts of fruit puree. If these agree with the baby, the amount can be increased to twice 1 oz. (30g) daily. From the twelfth week, the carrot juice can be replaced by mashed carrot.

During the fourth month the fruit puree can be mixed with rusk, or raw grated apple mixed with mashed banana can be given. Thus during the fifth and sixth month a breast-fed baby will be having four feeds from the breast and in addition a mid-morning feed with mashed vegetable and an afternoon feed with fruit puree.

What if the baby refuses the breast?

Some newborn babies, especially those who are premature, are too weak to suck. They can be fed on milk obtained from the mother with a breast pump. Indeed, more than any, these weak or premature babies need their own mother's milk.

Babies with deformed jaws, for instance a cleft palate, are also unable to suck from the breast and they too can be fed on mother's milk drawn off with a pump. These babies often have a tenacious will to live and thrive almost without help.

Any noticeable clumsiness in sucking should be pointed out to the doctor, who should also be consulted if the baby is consistently lazy about drinking.

If the baby has once or twice been given a bottle with too large a hole in the teat he may refuse the breast because it demands more hard work. Or if he has a cold and a blocked nose he will keep trying to suck and then let go to breathe. (See *Colds*, page 90).

The baby may also refuse the breast if he and his mother are both too nervous and excitable. The mother will have to try and be more calm and take life more slowly and the doctor may have to help with a harmless sedative or a calming herb tea. With patience this situation can usually be overcome and the baby still be pursuaded to drink from the breast.

2. BOTTLE FEEDING

It is quite easy to increase a baby's weight considerably. But the real art of nutrition lies in avoiding any over-feeding. In cases of illness, overweight children are in greater danger than those with the correct weight.

What are bio-dynamic foods (Demeter)?

The realisation that modern agricultural methods were aimed one-sidedly at increasing the *quantity* of food available for the ever growing population of the earth, while *quality* was deteriorating alarmingly, led a number of farmers and gardeners to seek advice from Rudolf Steiner on how to care for soil, crops and live-stock in ways that would increase their health and quality rather than their quantity only. From these meetings the bio-dynamic method of agriculture and horticulture evolved, in which special attention is paid to the preparation of natural fertilisers and composts.

Grain, vegetables and fruit grown in accordance with these methods are of the highest quality. Doctors who have been advising their patients for years to use such produce know the beneficial effect on health and growth, while anyone eating them cannot fail to notice their superior flavour and quality. Recognised producers on the European continent use the brand name 'Demeter'. This and other names are also available in British health food shops.

Feeding with Demeter Holle Baby Food

This baby food is made from grain grown by the bio-dynamic method. After forty years' experience I can say without hesitation that its use with cows' milk guarantees the best possible development in babies. They drink, and later eat, it with obvious relish and their development shows that it is the best possible substitute for breast milk.

It is simple to use, but the following suggestions will enable mothers to exercise their responsibility and ingenuity with a degree of variation not possible with ordinary baby foods. In this way they can really enter into the way in which they feed their babies, and need take nothing for granted.

The number and timing of feeds and the amount per feed

On the whole the baby can be given as much as he

takes eagerly. Amazingly, when the food conforms to mother's milk as closely as possible, babies usually take to within 5g the amount they would have taken if fed at the breast. It is not necessary for the baby to drink exactly the same amount at each feed. But though it is good to be flexible about the amount, it is necessary to be quite strict about the number of meals and their timing. Demand feeding has its place only in the early days until the baby has found his own rhythm. It is a great help to the little organism if the feeds are given regularly at the same time and with the same intervals each day. This is particularly so with babies who are not breast-fed. During the early weeks, once a rhythm has been established, the baby will wake almost to the minute at the right time for each feed. So the mother will know that if he cries at other times there is something else the matter.

Generally it is found that most babies feed at 6 a.m., 10 a.m., 2 p.m., 6 p.m. and 10 p.m. or thereabouts. Consideration for the child's freedom must not be exaggerated to the extent that the baby becomes a small despot. However, from time to time it will become plain that an adjustment of the daily rhythm has fallen due.

FOR THE PREPARATION OF THE MILK AND HOLLE CEREAL MIXTURE SEE APPENDIX THREE, P.208.

Bottle feeding during the first month

On the first day give only a few teaspoons of fennel tea. Proper feeding starts on the second day with five feeds of about ⅔oz. (20g) of milk and water (half and half).

On the third day feeding with the Holle mixture begins. However, in the case of babies weighing less than 6½lbs (3000g) at birth and those who are not very robust it is best to start with Demeter wheat or oat flakes in place of the Holle No.1 mixture for the first four weeks, and to go over to Holle No.1. in the fifth week. (Holle No.2 can be started in about the fourth month.)

Average babies are offered five feeds of about 1 oz. (25 to 30g) of Holle No.1 mixture on the third day. After this a daily increase of up to ⅓oz. (5 to 10g) per feed continues till the tenth day, when five feeds of about 3 oz. (80g) each are given.

From the end of the second week the amounts given on page 98 for breast feeding apply, with the exception of premature or otherwise ailing babies.

Bottle feeding during the second month

If the baby's mixture has so far been with Demeter oats or wheat flakes, now is the time for the changeover to a mixture made with Holle Baby Food No.1., which is made from bio-dynamically grown oats, wheat and rye made easily digestible by a special process. Many babies already thrive on this mixture during the first month, but it is too heavy for some to start with (see above).

Bottle feeding during the third month

The amount given can be increased gradually, but should not exceed 800g daily for an average baby. At the same time the transition can be made from the half and half Holle No. 1 mixture to the two thirds Holle

No. 1 mixture (See Appendix Three, p.208) by giving the thicker mixture for an additional feed every two days until all the feeds are made with this. If sufficient weight increase is not achieved with 28 oz. (800g) per day, the amounts for the fourth month can be given towards the end of the third month.

So by the end of the third month the baby will be having 4 or 5 bottle feeds. In addition he may have small amounts of mashed raw fruit, particularly grated apple, and also carrot juice and Weleda or Wala elixirs of wild fruits (Cranberry, Blackthorn, Rowan, Rose Hip).

Bottle feeding during the fourth month

The changeover to Holle Baby Food No.2 can now begin and like all changes in diet it should take place slowly. First the new mixture is used for one feed only. Two days later a second feed is changed over, and so on until all feeds are of Baby Food No.2, which is a whole grain food. After this the amount of milk can also be increased until the daily amount is about 21 oz. (600g) milk, 14 oz. (400g) Baby Food No.2. and seven or eight teaspoons of sugar divided into five feeds of 6½ to 7 oz. (180 to 200g) each.

Average babies change over to 4 meals a day during the fourth month and start on more solid food. A typical day's meal would be: 6-7 a.m. a two thirds mixture of Baby Food No.2; 11 a.m. increasing amounts of vegetables (carrots, spinach), followed by a bottle of Baby Food No.2., two thirds mixture (7 oz or 200g if the baby is having 4 meals a day); during the afternoon, 3 p.m., increasing amounts of mashed fruit followed again by a bottle of Baby Food No.2; in the evening, 6 p.m. repeat of the morning feed, or start to give a pap made from Baby Food No.2.

Feeding during the fifth month

The milky meals remain as for the fourth month. The afternoon meal can be augmented by mashing two rusks with the stewed fruit. The mid-day vegetable feed is also increased to a proper meal. If the baby refuses vegetables, mix them with some fruit.

There is no need to worry about over-eating. Hardly any child of this age will eat more than eight to ten dessertspoons of mixed vegetables and fruit.

In winter and spring several dessertspoons of fresh fruit juice may be added to the vegetable mixture immediately before feeding, but remember that fast electric mixers and also simply exposure to air destroy vitamins.

Most babies will now be having four meals a day, so that the last meal can be at 8 p.m. or sooner. The longer sleep during the night partly replaces nourishment, so that the bottle feeds need only be increased by about 1 oz. (20 to 30g).

Feeding from the sixth to the ninth month

The child now starts to need more and more solid food. Bottle feeds can be reduced to two a day, or from the eighth month one bottle feed in the morning and a milky pudding in the evening. During the eighth month, the transition can be made from two thirds milk to undiluted milk for the mixture. One of the meals now consists entirely of vegetables and another of a mixture of mashed fruit and rusk. Each meal is about 7 oz. (200g). The vegetables are also mixed with grain products, e.g. flakes of various kinds. Some butter may be added, or a little unheated oil, and possibly a pinch of sugar.

If the child is thirsty, specially during the summer, give him weak fennel, camomile or yarrow tea.

Extra fruit should be given before the meal, especially before the milk pudding. Thus the evening meal can consist of fruit followed by the milk pudding, or milk pudding mixed with rusk or curd cheese. The child can be given a biscuit, rusk or crust of wholemeal bread to nibble at by himself.

Suitable vegetables are carrots, spinach, cooked lettuce, young kohlrabi, cauliflower and tomatoes. This makes considerable variety possible. The choice of vegetables and grains should depend on the nature of the individual child.

(See *Some considerations when choosing food* page 112).

Feeding from the tenth to the twelfth month
By about the ninth month many children already have two more more teeth, but whether they have teeth or not, now is the time for them to learn to chew. If the gums are very sore with teething then wait a little, but otherwise start giving small cubes of bread with butter and honey or some good jam. The further development of the jaws and also the maintenance of healthy teeth have a great deal to do with sufficient chewing. So from

this age and continuing right through childhood it is good to ensure that children do enough proper chewing by giving them every day a thick piece or crust of hard, stale whole-grain bread which demands strenuous chewing.

Milk can now be given undiluted, but it is still more digestible if it is diluted, perhaps with a little grain coffee. The daily amount should still not exceed about a pint.

The child can of course now join the family at table for some or all meals, but he should not yet share the adults' diet, which is still too rich in protein. Once he has tasted eggs, meat and sausage he will start refusing his own more suitable but less interesting diet.

Curd cheese thinned with a little milk and mixed with any fruit in season is an excellent dish for the child's evening meal. Care should be taken to ensure that the cheese is of good quality. Alternatives are semolina pudding with fruit or rusks soaked in fruit juice. The amount can be up to 200 or 300g and the child should be really satisfied.

3. MILK-FREE DIET FOR BABIES

A mother whose baby is allergic to cows' milk and who herself has insufficient breast milk is faced with a considerable problem, especially if her doctor sees no way round starting the child too early on meat and eggs as an alternative. Many mothers will feel instinctively that this is not the solution.

A homoeopathic preparation made by Weleda from

potentised cows' milk is now available. It is found that the allergy often disappears after a single dose of a few drops, provided that it is a genuine milk allergy. In the case of an allergy to the mother's milk, the preparation can be made from her milk, even if she herself is strongly allergic. The allergic eczema starts to heal immediately, usually on the same day, and never erupts again. This success is achieved even if the child is not fed on a milk-free diet.

However, there are children who are not cured by this preparation. In these cases almond milk has been shown by Dr. M.E. Bircher, the esteemed dietary reformer, to be a suitable substitute. Rudolf Steiner also recommended it as a fully adequate substitute for milk. Babies only a few days old can be fed with it, whereby even nutritional diseases are healed.

Alternatively, baby food made from soya beans (obtainable from health food shops) may help. This is also effective in treating cystitis and pyelonephritis in the child. These complaints can be very stubborn in babies.

Chapter Nine

SOME GENERAL POINTS ABOUT FEEDING CHILDREN

Diet as the child grows older

Children of a year and older gradually cut more and more teeth and therefore should do more and more chewing. They can now be given bread for breakfast and for the afternoon meal, good whole grain or crisp bread, never white. Good jam and honey with this should help satisfy the child's need for sweet things. If the mother cannot prevent people from giving her children sweets and chocolate, she should at least take these into her care and dole them out very sparingly, perhaps as a reward when the child's pants are dry, etc. Sucking sweets must never be allowed to become a habit. It is not only the teeth that suffer. The stomach and the nervous system can also be affected because too much sugar can cause a vitamin B1 deficiency.

Suitable savoury spreads are cream cheese or other mild soft cheeses. Sharply seasoned meat pastes and sausages are not suitable till much later, especially as most types of sausage usually contain a good deal of pork.

If after careful consideration it is decided to give the child meat, then in the early years only the white meat of young animals should be used. Broth is of no great value for children, though if slightly anaemic a child will benefit from time to time from broth made from veal bones.

It is well worth going into the matter of giving children cereal products instead of meat. All kinds of muesli and also porridges made from various whole grains are suitable. It is a good idea to buy these whole and grind them oneself just before use. The various whole grain flakes (Demeter or Holle if possible) such as oats, barley and wheat are useful as a dish on their own when soaked in milk or juice. Highly processed cereal products such as cornflakes or puffed wheat are not recommended.

Whole grain foods of the kind just mentioned are also useful in encouraging lazy children to chew properly. The same can be said of almonds, hazel nuts and walnuts, which are also rich in protein and fats.

Yogurt with or without fruit is also a good food for children as are butter milk and home-made sour milk. As regards yogurt it should be remembered, however, that it is one of the foods invented by sheep and cattle herding tribes whose staple diet is meat. It has been found that if eaten in large quantities by vegetarians it can upset the stomach bacteria. So care should be taken with yogurt given to small children before meat has been introduced into their diet.

When children start sharing the adults' meals, care should be taken that the food does not contain vinegar (except cider vinegar), pepper, mustard or too much salt. Salad dressings should be made with sour cream or lemon and oil. Herbs, dried or fresh, added to vegetables in small quantities are quite acceptable. Fresh herbs are even better than dried; they stimulate the digestive glands and help keep away colds of all kinds.

If the child persists in rejecting a new food, the mother can do her best to demonstrate with words and gestures how delicious it is. For all normal foods there is no harm in applying a little gentle force if the child is not even prepared to try, for instance some new vegetable. Rather than distracting him with toys or the radio it is better to let him go hungry for one or two meals and he will then at least condescend to try what he is offered. If he still does not like it then return to other vegetables and try again a week or two later.

Spinach has a high content of oxalic acid and nitrate and can therefore be dangerous for small babies. It should never be warmed up for them after the first cooking, and where possible bio-dynamic quality only should be used.

Some considerations when choosing food

Meat and eggs are quite superfluous for babies. Milk has plenty of protein and later curd cheese can also be added to meals several times a week. In rare cases a baby will occasionally need half an egg yolk towards the end of his first year, and this should be from a very fresh egg. Meat and broth are only necessary if the milk, cereals and other foods are of a very poor quality. If Holle and Demeter or other similar good foods are given, there need be no anxiety about the adequacy of the baby's diet.

Most potato varieties are today degenerating, so that they cannot be recommended for little children. Even as adults we feel rather dull if we have eaten too many potatoes. For children this is more far-reaching because potatoes are not good for the development of the brain. Unpolished natural rice is the best substitute for potatoes whenever possible. Millet is also good. But of course there is no harm in children eating a certain amount of potatoes, though they should never have them in the evening.

It is medically recognised that coffee, tea, alcohol and all cola drinks are totally undesirable until after puberty.

Chapter Ten

UPBRINGING

Early training

It has been said that we are living in the century of the child, and many parents and teachers feel that it is wrong to 'interfere with the child's freedom'. This is a complete misunderstanding of what a child needs and expects from parents and teachers alike. The very way in which he explores how far he can take naughtiness, disobedience, destructiveness and lack of respect shows that he is seeking definite guidance.

During the very early years, when he is building himself and his world through observation and imitation, he needs adults to set him an example.

Then, when he ceases to call himself by name but starts to say 'I', he begins to be aware of himself, and in order to experience himself he must of necessity come up against his surroundings. At the height of this phase he says 'no' to everything. If he is not answered with unambiguous commands he is deeply disappointed in the depths of his being and feels driven to repeated experimental provocative action.

If the child encounters the laws of nature by burning his fingers or hurting himself in some other way, then these very laws reprimand and teach him through the pain he experiences. But moral or ethical laws must be represented by mature human beings who reprimand him when he transgresses against them, for these higher laws do not protect themselves, and the child should not

be allowed to go against them uncorrected. Through
words and deeds which are in keeping with the child's
comprehension the adults around him must make it
clear what is and what is not done. There is no hiding
behind high principles from laziness.

With very small children rules and prohibitions of
course go in at one ear and out at the other. During the
earlier years the child has to be shown his limits by the
tone of voice and consistence. Often it is more a matter
of distracting his attention to something else rather
than trying to establish a rule he cannot yet understand.
But even an eighteen-month-old is quite capable of
learning what is 'dirty' or 'hot', though he cannot be
protected from all bad experiences. The main thing is to
keep him safe from serious harm.

It is most important in bringing up children to avoid
being uncertain and anxious. This is simply annoying
for a healthy child and is in itself a temptation to
defiance, whereas for a sick child it is a burden that
disturbs and even prevents him from getting well.

The child's urge to be active

There are divergent opinions about the degree to
which children should be hemmed in during their early
years. In western countries the tendency is to leave
them almost entirely free. The consequence of this
seems to be increasingly wild and almost despotic behaviour by children who almost terrorise their families,
visitors and even neighbours till finally the exasperated
parents see nothing for it but to dump them in front of
the television screen to keep them quiet.

Children are left excessively free out of a kind of sentimental misunderstanding of what a child needs from those who bring him up. In fact neither unlimited freedom to fidget and rush about nor too much restriction is good for the child. As with everything, the happy medium has to be found. For considerations regarding the balance between firm wrapping and letting the small baby kick, see page 92.

As the child continues to grow, the proper use of the playpen or walker will be the next question to crop up. This useful apparatus can be damaging if seen simply as a means of curbing the annoying fidgetiness of an active child or if it is used to imprison a child who is too old. But with proper use it gives the baby for a few hours a day a little realm of his own, while freeing his mother from having to keep a watchful eye on him every minute of his waking hours. Efforts have been made to make less cage-like play-pens (Heilinstitut Schloss Bingenheim, Post Friedberg/Land, West Germany).

Rocking is another important element in upbringing. A baby rocked in a cradle for his first few months is most unlikely to grow into a child who later has the habit of sitting up in bed in the evening or even in the middle of the night rocking to and fro to the accompaniment of his own rhythmical sing-song. Later, nothing could be better than a hammock, rocking chair or rocking horse to satisfy his fundamental need for rhythmical movement. In contrast, the bouncing chairs and seats now available on the market go against the natural swinging rhythm of breathing. The child's obvious enjoyment of this bouncing movement is not necessarily the only criterion, for he will anyway delight in any kind of motion and activity.

Reins and harness are excellent for curbing an active child out in the streets and lend themselves perfectly to 'horsey' games.

So, give the child freedom to move about and be active within normal limits, and he will not need periods of wild romping and rushing that do him no good. There will be a period when nothing will be safe from him and he will need constant supervision, but this is unavoidable. Later he will continue to satisfy his need to move by climbing about on the apparatuses in children's playgrounds, and with his scooter, tricycle, or toboggan in winter. When he is five or six he will learn to swim. (It is an exaggeration of a good idea to teach babies to swim).

Play

For children, play is pure artistry and serves no practical purpose. When they are undisturbed by adults they are genial and take little account of detail. Indeed, a small child who places his building bricks exactly and neatly one upon the other is not playing; he is likely to become pedantic to no small degree. It is not good to disturb a child who is absorbed in a game of his own, specially not to give him adult advice about how his play should proceed. On the other hand, if he wants to tell you about his games, listen seriously and do not criticise or make out your superiority. A child's games are like beautiful dreams and their influence will remain with him all his life.

Do not be surprised or upset when the oldest and shabbiest teddy is more beloved than the beautiful new doll. Try to arrange with grandparents and godparents what presents should be given so that the child is not submerged in toys. And if he has too many, hide some for a while and let them appear again later on.

Free painting on white paper with water colours (not filling in pre-drawn pictures!) is a most satisfying artistic play activity, as is modelling with coloured wax.

When the child goes to school, the concentration he has learned through undisturbed play will stand him in good stead and he will be ready to accept with gratitude and attention the suggestions and ideas of the teacher, especially if these are given in an artistic way. It is best to wait at least till he starts school before giving the child mechanical toys, and it is to be hoped that fathers who long for electric trains will wait till their boys are about ten years old.

Far more damage than is realised is done by allowing children to embark too early on a new phase.

So-called bad habits

A number of so-called 'bad habits' in children are nothing more than imitation or a game and should not be judged from a moral standpoint. 'Thefts' of money or trinkets, nibbling food or sweets on the sly, taking toys and other objects to pieces, are all things that can be dealt with by understanding parents and teachers. Even tormenting or killing insects and worms is probably no more than a misplaced desire to explore the world. Parents and teachers could do well to seek the origin of the 'bad habit' in their own behaviour. Certainly they should try to think with the child rather than against him in order to get to the bottom of what might be causing the problem. Once they have found the cause, gentle guidance and understanding will usually be sufficient to bring it to an end.

Similarly when little children play with their genitals it is nonsense to talk of masturbation. A bored child left sitting on the potty for too long is quite likely to fiddle about, but there is no more to this than if he were to pick his nose or bite his nails. If the parents react with horror and indignation, however, the child will start to have all sorts of suspicions. So instead of smacking or scolding, simply give him something else to do with his hands, just as you would quietly persist in removing his thumb from his mouth again and again when trying to break the thumb-sucking habit. Also avoid leaving him on the potty for too long in the first place and see that he does not lie awake for hours in bed. Inflammation of the genitals arising from a chill or the rubbing of tight clothes can also turn the child's attention too much in that direction.

The facts of life

Up to as late as the tenth year a child's questions about his origin are concerned fundamentally with his spiritual origins. The facts of physical conception and birth only become really comprehensible when the ability to observe objectively and think abstractly starts to develop. Thus early explanations and, worse still, practical demonstrations completely miss the point and show a total misunderstanding of the child's being and development.

The small child is non-sexual. Interest and understanding for sexual processes starts to emerge with the onset of puberty between the ages of 12 and 15 years. Parallel with it the young person's own moral capacities and thought life begin to awaken. Till then he lives more within the feelings and ideas of those around him. Thus the examples set by uninhibited sensuality or sensible and serious behaviour will have definite effects on the way he enters and copes with puberty and his awakening sexual urges.

Other aspects that affect the onset of puberty lie much earlier on in the child's life. Overfeeding, especially with eggs and meat, causes infants to lose their childlike qualities and grow up too quickly, and later on puberty is likely to be early and difficult. For the same reason pepper, paprika, mustard and vinegar, and even too much salt, are unsuitable in the diet of small children. Overstimulation of the senses, e.g. constant background noise from radio and television, glaring and overbright decor in the child's surroundings accompanied by too many toys, too many different new foods and tastes all at once, all this causes children to mature physically more quickly than they should, which in turn means that puberty arrives before the child's mental and emotional development can cope with it.

Bed wetting

By the age of two-and-a-half the child should be clean

and dry by day and night. A proper relationship between waking and sleeping is established, and this in turn determines the excretory functions. Constant wetting by day and night can have many causes. The child may have a bladder complaint, or simply a chill caused by insufficient warm clothing for the lower half of his body. Or there may be a psychological problem such as jealousy of siblings, definite fears, environmental disturbances, etc. In most cases the doctor will be able to assist either with medicaments (Weleda) or with advice. When the bed wetting stops, there will also be positive effects on the child's soul life and development.

Fear and anxiety

Most of us will remember the fears suffered during childhood, the fear of dogs and other animals, caterwauling in the garden at night that we took for the crying of children, creaking noises in furniture and floors, or even fear of certain people.

Fear is often occasioned by noises that are not understood or by the first inklings of animal urges and instincts. Often also children tune in to the existential fear that afflicts so many adults these days.

Strangely enough, the fears experienced by children during bombing raids in the last war appear to have left no noticeable psychological scars. But it seems that the shocks had a direct influence on the life forces themselves, for many people have subsequently come to suffer physically from a marked constitutional weakness. Fear disturbs the building up processes and cramps the blood vessels.

Often the doctor only hears about a child's fears by chance during consultations about 'proper' illnesses. This is partly because parents know from experience that they are likely to be given nothing more than a sedative, which they instinctively feel will not do the child any good. Or they may be under the impression that psychological problems cannot be helped with medicines. Thus many children suffer agonies for years when they could quite well be helped by the doctor.

Unfortunately many parents still bring up their children with the help of hints about the 'bogey man' or some other threatening character. Fears can also arise as a result of television or radio programmes, or even a visit to a circus or the zoo. Children cannot absorb too many impressions, especially those which are incomprehensible to their childish understanding. These undigested experiences then reappear in their dreams. Even an evening meal that is too heavy can cause nightly fears.

If a child has a nightmare, make sure that he wakes up fully, if necessary by wiping his face with a cold sponge. He will then usually go to sleep again quite peacefully after a comforting chat. If there is anything that frightens him, remove it if possible. Often a dim lamp in the bedroom does wonders.

But if the child is not comforted by ordinary means, a doctor should definitely be consulted. Sometimes childhood fears can lead to neuroses later.

Radio and television
Some people feel that even small babies need

constant background music from the radio. Later they allow their children to do their homework while the radio is on. Some children are so addicted that they imagine they cannot even do their homework unless the radio is blaring. And the television has encroached even further on social and family life, to the extent that it often determines daily routine.

Daily doses of television work on the child in the following way: A profusion of scenes that cannot possibly be assimilated psychologically pass before his eyes in rapid succession. (The impact made by colour television is even more startling, i.e. red blood is bloodier than black blood). School work begins to suffer, not necessarily because the children are distracted from finishing their homework and go to bed too late, but because the agitating rapid sequence of pictures occasions a high degree of physical fidgetiness. Moreover, soul activity and creativity of will remain underdeveloped.

It is now known that television can cause a number of serious medical conditions: damage to eyes and ears, heart and circulatory disturbances (TV angina pectoris); and above all postural damage (TV neck). Latent epilepsy can also be activated. A number of hospitals now have special departments in their paediatric clinics for TV damaged children.

If a child's tummy is upset through the consumption of food that disagrees with him, steps are taken to make sure that he does not eat the same dish again. Yet if a child's constitution is spoilt by radio and television this is not even noticed, mainly because people are not aware that this is a possibility. Often the disturbance and damage is indeed not very noticeable, but it is serious because the child's physical organs are still being completed as he grows, and their ultimate delicacy or grossness is largely dependent on the sense impressions to which he is subject during this process.

Pre-school learning — a disaster

For a number of years now pre-school learning has been described as representing a decisive advantage by educationalists intent on being progressive. They say that children both can and want to start learning much earlier, that their ability to learn is particularly great during the first four years and that by the fourth year 50% of their intelligence is either developed or lost for ever. They hold that talent is not something with which children are born but that they can be educated to have it and that as the social environment is more important than heredity one must start early to promote intellectual capacity by giving the children stimulating tasks.

None of these statements is absolutely wrong and they are a good example of how half-truths are often more dangerous and difficult to shift than outright errors or lies. They are based on the opinion that hitherto the faculties of three- to five-year-old children have been wasted and that they are insufficiently educated if they have not been taught to read from the age of three.

It is really tragic that young politicians and young people in general, lacking as they are in life experience, make particularly extreme demands for experiments in pre-school learning. No doubt they have the best intentions but we have so far lost our healthy instincts today that it is not good enough to base actions solely on good will. Reform efforts of this kind must be based on very fundamental knowledge of the child's nature. The demands sound so obvious and seem quite logical but they completely disregard the real laws of child development.

We have all met examples of these precocious and prematurely old children and seen the way their ambitious parents show off their party tricks. In extreme cases they are infant prodigies who develop really spectacular achievements at a very early age. But follow them into later life and you will find that the overwhelming majority become pitiful creatures whose creative forces have all been exhausted in childhood. At best they become completely onesided specialists in some narrow field, not complete human beings able to think, feel and act harmoniously.

All parents can observe how a small baby cries with might and main, becoming bright red and really showing his fury. This strengthens his breathing. A little later they see how he practises tirelessly with his little hands, watching them as they move. Then he starts to kick, to pull himself up and to crawl. And finally he learns to walk and run about, falling often, picking himself up and running on, beaming with delight. He grows steadier, arms and legs come under control and his balance improves. He really works at becoming oriented in space. Soon his activities extend to his scooter and his tricycle and his arms are also used increasingly as he 'helps' his mother with her housework and copies every activity he sees around him. He tirelessly exercises his speech organs and the muscles which help him see and touch. In short, for the first seven years the child has an untameable primeval urge to be active in every possible way with his body.

Now it is essential to recognise that all this activity of limbs and all movable parts of the body including every muscle of the metabolic organs has one common denominator: the development of the will. All these activities are subject to the will, partly consciously and partly unconsciously. The stimulus for all movements, except reflex actions, comes from the will forces of the soul which in a way grasp the limbs from the outside and lead them to whatever the soul feels as a wish. Only muscles can actually move. The inner process of every movement is made possible by complicated metabolic processes which remain in the unconscious unless there are injuries or illnesses such as rheumatism. All kinds of movement are expressions of will.

So far we have described only the external aspect of movement. There is also an internal aspect which leads us into the most intimate part of man's being. Where is a person most himself? In thoughts and words he can dissemble or lie and give out knowledge he has read in books as his own creation. It is in his actions that he reveals his most intimate intentions. His acts of will reveal his personality and in the final analysis determine his destiny. Even consciously linking one thought to another is only possible through the will.

This is the depth and breadth required for understanding the development of the will life. And to develop all the possibilities of his will a child needs the first seven years of his life from birth until he changes his teeth. Every minute is filled to bursting with this process and not an instant is lost. Through ceaseless movement in the first seven years the will is developed.

However, this development can be disregarded and brought into disharmony. We can do gymnastics with a one-year-old or teach him to swim. Though this is too early for regimented movement, at least it is movement. But if we cause the child to use his intellectual capacities in reading and writing while he is still too young and should be developing his will through movement, we make him use up forces which are not yet mature and which later in life will be sorely lacking as a result. That many children enter happily into this kind of activity is no justification, for all children enjoy being at the centre of adult attention. It is also no excuse to say that we are not forcing the children but are leading them to reading and writing through play. Childish play should be entirely aimless and involve only the imagination and the will but not the intellect.

It will be the doctors who find themselves dealing with the consequences of pre-school learning. The surplus vitality needed by adults to cope with life and work in the world are used up in childhood so that the very opposite happens from the ideal imagined by the advocates of pre-school learning: ability and efficiency decrease instead of increasing. The beginning of this can be seen in the children themselves when they grow pale, sleep badly, grow slowly and tire easily. Conversely the results of a childhood without early learning and with plenty of time to develop the will properly can be seen in some of the grand old men of our time such as Churchill, Adenauer or Henry Ford who all had childhood days without the problems of early intellectual training.

One of the greatest fallacies of today is the belief that whatever is possible is also permissible; innumerable things are possible, but to do many of them is utter foolishness or worse.

Not only the will, but all three basic capacities of the soul develop according to fundamental laws. Just as the will needs the first seven years to develop properly, so the feeling life starts its real development when the child is of school age, while the thinking capacity develops fully last of all. Though all three are present from the start, they depend for their unfolding on a process of maturation undergone by the living formative forces mentioned so often in this book. And if these forces are used up before they are mature there is no going back and the relative soul forces are not fully developed.

So as far as the development of the will is concerned, what a child needs until the change of teeth is not pre-school training but a good kindergarten where his will forces can be developed in a meaningful way. His learning at this age is not intellectual but mainly the copying of physical actions.

The Sick Child

Chapter Eleven

THE SICK CHILD

1. GENERAL POINTS

What is illness?

Why should man, the pinnacle of creation, suffer from so many illnesses? If he were the same as any natural creation, stone, plant, animal, there would be no inner reasons for him to become ill. But because of his spiritual aspect, man is above nature, he is a citizen of both the natural and the spiritual world. He has developed beyond his links with nature and now lives in the conflict between the natural and the spiritual part of his total personality.

With his physical body and the etheric life forces working in it, he is more or less subject to the laws of the natural world. But with his soul and spirit he has separated himself from the life of nature. This inner contrast is the source of his special human capabilities and achievements, but it also contains the possibility of aberrations and mistakes, and of disturbances of inner harmony that are the cause of all illnesses. Man has achieved the ability to live and act in opposition to the ancient divine spiritual laws; he is on the way to achieving freedom of action, but he has to pay for this with the possibility of disease. Having lost his instinct for what is good and right, he has opened the door to sin, disease and death.

How does healing take place?

It is the anthroposophical doctor's task so to stimulate and strengthen the patient's life forces that the body can heal itself. This is indeed the aim of all healing and of the medicaments used.

There is a fundamental distinction, however, between the method of doctors who use medicaments derived from nature and those who use chemically synthetic medicines. A chemical medicament contains no living forces and it can therefore not stimulate a healing process, since dead materials cannot bring about living processes. A chemical medicament can, though, have chemical effects, for instance the dulling of pain or the killing of bacteria, but there is an accompanying danger of damage to the living forces. The anthroposophical and homoeopathic doctor uses preparations derived from natural animal, plant and mineral substances, and with these he is able to affect not only the physical body but also the life forces working in it. It is his aim to strengthen these forces to the extent that they can themselves take on the healing of the illness.

The healing power of fever

The ego, the spiritual centre of the personality, has already been mentioned a number of times as the force which welds together the other three members of man into a totality. The ego is the 'master of the house', keeping order and seeking to keep out intruders. But if something foreign, for instance poison, cold or bacteria, does manage to enter, the ego has to do battle. Its weapon is an increase in body temperature, in other words a fever. A fever brings about reactions and calls up all the life forces to the defence. The doctor can work with a fever and there are even means of bringing on a beneficial fever. The intruding foreign influence is 'digested' more thoroughly than food by means of the fever.

Thus the ego's efforts can be supported by the use of hot compresses, sweat treatment and baths and preparations that raise the body temperature. In the last resort, all efforts to restore order in the 'household' stem from the ego, with the resulting symptoms in the organism of the life forces. Thus so long as inflammation and temperature correspond with one another, there is no danger.

We should try to overcome our fear of heightened temperatures. Parents should never demand that the doctor give their child a medicine that suppresses fever, for fever is an integral part of many illnesses. Often a critical situation arises if there is no fever, or if it has been suppressed. There is no cause for concern when the state of the illness and the height of the temperature correspond with each other. I have twice met with children who were perfectly well three days after having had a temperature of 107.7°F (42.3°C).

2. ACUTE ILLNESSES

Birth damage

A newborn baby can have considerable swellings on his head resulting from the birth process. These are filled with liquid and can be quite large. They should be examined immediately, but are nearly always harmless and disappear rapidly, especially after the application of Mercurialis ointment (Weleda). Sometimes considerable growths remain, which disappear more slowly. Some swellings on the head are more serious, however.

On the other hand, the distortions of the skull that can come about during birth are nearly always quite harmless and disappear within a few days. Fortunately the individual bones of the skull are not yet firmly anchored and so can give way to the pressure. Parents need therefore not be alarmed if their baby's head displays a decidedly startling shape when they first see him. This will soon rectify itself.

If during the early weeks the baby is obviously clumsy about taking the breast or cannot seem to learn to take a proper hold, or if he is excessively passive, the doctor should be informed. There may be a brain haemorrhage, which is fairly frequent though rarely with lasting ill effects. If it is serious, the consequences are unconsciousness, cramps or unwillingness to drink.

The doctor should also be called if the baby's skin begins to turn yellow during the first day. 'Normal' jaundice of the newborn does not set in till the second or third day and usually disappears after two or three weeks. Premature babies retain the yellowish colouring longer, as do congenitally retarded children.

Not infrequently the baby's collar bone is broken during birth. Usually this mends by itself without treatment, but the doctor must decide whether anything should be done.

Ailments during the early months

There can be a swelling of the breast glands in both
boys and girls soon after birth as a result of hormonal
adjustment. This contains so-called 'lac neonatorum',
which should not be expelled from the breast by
squeezing. It is much better to leave the swelling alone
or apply Mercurialis ointment and it will disappear
quite soon.

Bleeding from the navel after the remainder of the
umbilical cord has been discarded can also cause
mothers anxiety, but this is quite harmless so long as
the navel has been kept scrupulously clean. The
bleeding can be stopped quite easily, for instance by
applying an arnica dressing (10 drops Weleda Arnica
20% in half a cup of water). The doctor will only have to
be called in rare cases.

Wild flesh sometimes grows in the navel making a
lump as big as a cherry stone or even a hazel nut. In this
case too, the doctor must be consulted. It is essential to
keep the navel absolutely clean until the wound is quite
healed. If despite these precautions there should be
signs of swelling, redness or dampness, or a bad smell or
pus, or a hernia or growth, the doctor must be consulted. Regarding umbilical and other hernias see next
section.

Newborn babies quite often have pink birthmarks of
different sizes, usually symmetrically situated on both
halves of the head, particularly on the forehead, the
eyelids, the nose, the back of the head and the back of
the neck. These are caused by an enlargement of blood
vessels and usually disappear before the child is fifteen

months old, though in the nape of the neck they sometimes remain longer. They are quite harmless and require no treatment.

Another kind of birthmark is more serious. These, too, are caused by an enlargement of blood vessels but they are thicker and resemble dark red sponges which empty when pressed and then fill again with blood. These are not present at birth but grow during the early months, sometimes at considerable speed. Rapid growths of this kind can be dangerous and should be under constant observation. Recent research in America has shown that the rapid growth of these birthmarks usually ceases about the tenth month, though in some cases it continues till the child is two or more. Then they gradually disappear by themselves leaving only a hardly noticeable coloration of the skin by the time the child is six. This happens even if the birthmarks are large and thick. So parents should not urge the doctor to treat these marks, for no known methods have such good cosmetic results as self-healing. On the contrary, they lead to more or less permanent scarring. Since these marks are often on the face or other visible parts it takes courage to wait, but it is worth it.

Other birthmarks, brown or black moles with or without hairs, are said to be the result of the mother receiving a shock during pregnancy. If this were so, what should the babies have looked like who were born to mothers who went through the horrors of the blitz while pregnant!

The neck muscles are sometimes damaged during

birth, and the baby will then bend his head towards the painful side. Usually this will heal on its own, but occasionally the baby's head remains bent to one side. Usually this can be remedied with massage and applications of Mercurialis ointment, but just occasionally a small operation is necessary.

If forceps are used during the birth, this sometimes damages some of the facial muscles. The baby's mouth will then be crooked when he cries, or perhaps one eyelid will not close properly. The arm nerves can also be damaged, but this nearly always heals of its own accord.

Phimosis is quite common in infant boys. This is a narrowing of the foreskin which can cause difficulty in passing water. Usually the doctor can correct this during the early weeks by stretching. The foreskin finally stretches by itself during puberty.

In baby girls there is sometimes bleeding or a sticky discharge from the vagina. Like the breast swelling this is probably hormonal in origin and it is quite harmless, ceasing after a few days.

Hernias

The most common of these is the umbilical hernia. The navel sometimes does not heal properly when the remains of the umbilical cord have fallen away. A round, usually hard, lump is felt under the skin and can be easily pressed back into the tummy. However, when the baby cries or presses when passing a motion it is liable to pop out again and the hole tends to stretch, so that the lump can reach the size of a walnut or even more.

Above and below the navel, hernias of the abdominal wall can also occur. In the embryo, the abdominal wall grows together from both sides, but sometimes it does not knit together sufficiently in the middle, so that a slit is left open. A portion of the intestines can become pinched in this, which is very painful.

In less serious cases only the external skin bulges. Gentle pressure pushes the air back into the abdomen and the bulge disappears.

In both cases the doctor will apply a sticking plaster to hold the place closed in a fold of skin. This enables the weak part to shrink and grow together. Take care to dry the plaster well after bathing, as it should remain for some time. If necessary replace it with a fresh one. The small baby may need the plaster for three to four months. But if the hernia occurs later than eight or nine months the plaster method is no longer effective. The child will then need a small operation later.

On the whole umbilical hernias are not dangerous, although specially with girls they must be properly healed in view of the strain placed on the wall of the abdomen in pregnancy later on. Inguinal hernias (in the groin) can be much more serious, especially in boys, where intestines can be pushed right down into the scrotum, leading sometimes to strangulation of the intestine.

When a child cries with pain and cannot be soothed it is possible that the cause may be a hernia of this kind. Examine the groin on both sides. There will be a hard lump painful to the touch and the baby will cry continuously and keep stretching his legs. Place the baby in a warm bath or apply damp warm compresses to the swelling. If this does not cause the hernia to retract, the doctor must be called immediately, even in the middle of the night. The strangulation must not be allowed to continue for more than six hours. The doctor will probably be able to press the protruding part back into the abdomen, which immediately removes the pain as well as the danger. If he is unsuccessful the child will have to have an early operation. But quite often the bumping of the car on the way to the hospital causes the hernia to slip back.

Even tiny babies can be operated on if the hernia is acute, but it is better to wait till the child is more than a year old, using a rubber truss till then. In very thin children the hernia can close as a result of a rapid increase in weight, which can be achieved with a change of diet. Hernias in the groin are far more frequent in boys than in girls.

Rickets — history and incidence

Rickets occurs when there is insufficient assimilation of sunlight resulting in insufficient transformation of the provitamin in the skin into vitamin D. In consequence the organism fails to absorb sufficient mineral salts, especially calcium, from the food eaten. The bones and connective tissues remain soft and watery, there is bending of some bones and enlargement at the ends of others, for instance the knobbed appearance of the ribs where they join the cartilage of the breast bone. The bones at the back of the skull can become soft and flattened. And lack of tissue firmness in lungs and other internal organs weakens their functioning and gives the tendency for catarrhal complaints, diarrhoea and other afflictions. Directly connected with this delay in mineralisation of the body is a slowness of soul development: grasping, sitting, standing, speaking, and thinking are not achieved at the normal rate.

As a whole the disease can be characterised as a retardation of the incarnation of the formative forces of the soul and spirit, or as a retention of embryonic forms and qualities.

In the mid-twenties Professor Windaus developed artificial vitamin D and this led to a fundamental change in the rickets situation as it existed then. In some countries a prophylactic treatment was developed consisting of a few massive doses of vitamin D administered to babies during the early weeks of life. The effect was a spectacular hardening of the bones and connective tissues and it seemed as if the rickets problem was solved for good. Anyone trying to point out the disadvantages of this treatment was shouted down.

My own negative attitude to it began in the very early days of its application when I conducted an autopsy on a baby. I found that it had died from arteriosclerosis, a disease of old age.

In the months during which I was engaged with this case my medical thinking was influenced in a particular way. I came to the following conclusion: Human life flows like a river which is bound by certain laws and certain periodic developments during which specific advances take place. The baby learns to grasp, to sit, to

stand, to speak, to think and so on. Then comes the
middle period of life, and finally old age with its characteristic symptoms. Here, however, was a baby who had
died from a disease of advancing age. I realised that the
speed of life's stream can be altered and that it is not
necessarily bound to rigid laws.

As time went on it became more and more apparent
that large and even small doses of vitamin D were
leading to the permanent illness or death of numberless
children. An extensive literature is now available on the
subject and in most countries the treatment has been
discontinued in favour of a much longer treatment with
very small doses.

There are, however, still some who favour the
massive dose treatment, saying that mothers are too
neglectful and will not persist in administering small
doses over a long period. This may be true in a few
cases, but to most mothers it is an insult. And even if a
few are negligent, this is no reason for continuing such a
dangerous treatment across the board.

The symptoms of vitamin D poisoning are initially
constipation, followed by persistent lack of appetite and
slowing down of development, vomiting, headache,
hardening of the bones, kidney failure. The symptoms
are usually at their worst thirty to sixty days after the
dose has been administered.

In my opinion there is yet another aspect to be considered in this matter. The too rapid and too concen-
trated mineralisation of the child's body brought about
by massive dose treatment is accompanied by a
speeding up of the rest of the child's development. Just

as the body grows old too soon, so consciousness awakes too rapidly. To the misguided joy of some parents the children are precociously forward by the time they go to school. Many, however, begin to fall behind by the time they are ten or twelve. Though physically robust and often astonishingly tall, they fail in intellectual ability and teachers complain of lack of concentration, inattentiveness, nervous fidgetiness and lack of interest. Consciousness becomes narrowed down to a few specialised subjects and there is difficulty in thinking. There are, of course, also other factors which speed up the development of children today, in particular the ever growing influence of technology all around us.

In recent years the rickets cases seen by doctors have not only once again increased in number but have also become more serious than they have been for a long time and are sometimes combined with symptoms of tetany. The reasons for the increase and the accompanying symptoms are not exactly known, but it is my conviction that a decisive role is played by the increase in the amount of unsuitable foods given to babies: dried milk products, farinaceous products with no nutritional value, and tinned vegetables. Fortunately the disease is now never as extreme as it used to be.

Every newborn baby, even if breast-fed, is in danger of contracting rickets. Some are particularly susceptible, for instance babies whose mothers are particularly anaemic or suffer from calcium deficiency, babies born during the dark winter months, and also premature or weak babies. There are also families with an inherited tendency for rickets. Overfed babies and those fed mainly on dried milk products are also more in danger. Furthermore, the haze of pollution over industrial towns has now reached a stage where on many days the sun's ultraviolet rays can hardly penetrate through to the earth.

Rickets — *prevention and treatment*

So many requests have reached me from worried parents all over the world who know the dangers of vitamin D that I have decided to give in detail my method of preventing and treating rickets based on anthroposophical medicine. But parents should if possible consult their own doctor first. Perhaps he could read this section and then adjust the treatment to the individual case. They should also take the child to see him about once a month while the treatment lasts.

As has been said, rickets is becoming more frequent and virtually every child could contract the disease. Therefore prevention should start as early as five or six weeks. This applies particularly when the parents themselves have suffered from rickets, but also if the child is born in the winter months when there is little daylight or if the family lives in rather dark accommodation.

It must be stated categorically that treatment with calcium alone, even with the otherwise excellent Weleda Calcium Supplements I and II, is not a sufficiently dependable preventive method.

Even breast-fed babies can contract rickets, though the danger is far smaller than with bottle-fed infants. For the latter the advice on nutrition given in this book, particularly concerning the use of Demeter and Holle products, is especially important for the prevention of rickets. Over-feeding increases the probability of the disease.

It is important to remember that the illness is caused by lack of sunlight which can be considerable today in towns permanently covered by a haze of atmospheric pollution. Phosphorous can increase the effects of the available sunlight or act as a substitute when it is lacking. This is given in a homoeopathic potency, usually D6. Starting at about the fifth week, give the baby three drops morning and midday in a little water. Continue for four to six weeks and then pause for a week or a fortnight. In addition to this it is important to give in the morning a small saltspoon of calcium phosphate (apatite D6 or calcium phosphoricum D6) and in the evening a saltspoon of calcium carbonate (conchae verae D10 or calcium carbonicum D10). All these are given before meals in a little water.

In special cases cod-liver oil continues to prove useful. Choose a brand which is pure and natural and give the child one teaspoon twice daily if it does not upset his digestion.

In the case of rickety children whose parents have also suffered from the disease it is essential that they be taken to the doctor, if possible one who works with biological methods. In those who have inherited the illness even massive dose treatment with vitamin D has been known to fail. It is a matter of treating the whole constitution of the child with all possible biological methods.

A final cure of rickets takes time to achieve. Parents must therefore be patient, for it is not only a matter of a lack of solidity in the bones but also one of a disturbance in the process of incarnation. This tendency to develop too slowly must be overcome gently and not by force. In recent years it has frequently been stated in the relevant literature that a mild affliction of rickets need not be feared nearly as much as the danger of kidney, brain or heart disease caused by synthetic vitamin D. Certainly the opposite of rickets, an artificial speeding up of the development and excessive hardening of the bones together with a tendency to arterio-sclerosis, is a threat to health and strength which will follow a person throughout life. Conversely, rickets, except in serious or neglected cases, can be overcome during childhood with suitable treatment and then very rarely leaves a residue of bone deformation.

Apart from the above treatment with medicine, which it is up to the mother to carry out carefully and punctually, there are further possibilities for maintaining the child's health. The child's food must be of the best possible quality and contain enough natural vitamins and above all plenty of minerals. The Demeter and Holle products described in this book have proved excellent as aids to rickets prevention. It is essential for the baby to have gruels and puddings made with cereals and later to eat whole grain bread. A child with a large fontanel and other indications of rickets will need root vegetables and their raw juices, particularly carrots, from about the fourth month.

Another aid in preventing rickets is plenty of fresh air

and sunlight or outdoor daylight if the sun is not shining. In winter if it is windy and rather cold it is sufficient to take the child out for half or quarter of an hour. If a balcony or garden is available the child can be left out in his pram for hours if he is well wrapped up and tucked in with a hot water bottle. Strong east winds are dangerous however.

In the summer the child can be out of doors much longer and when this is not possible his cot should be placed directly beside the open window. On hot days he can be placed naked in the sun for a short while, first about two minutes on his back and two on his tummy. This can be gradually increased to about fifteen minutes. It is pointless to aim for a sun tan as quickly as possible because brown skin keeps the sun's rays out. Also it is important to remember that as a general rule the head, that is the brain and the spinal fluid, must not have too much sun, if only because this can favour the development of polio.

The value of a canopy of light red material (see page 78) has already been mentioned. This protects the baby from the inflammatory rays of the sun while letting through those which help prevent rickets. So under such a canopy the baby can be given much more sunlight than would be possible without.

Finally there are bath mixtures which help combat rickets. Those containing thyme are specially useful. Sulphur bath mixtures (Weleda or others) can also be used if available. These are given 3 times per week in courses of twelve baths.

Diarrhoea

Diarrhoea is rare in breast-fed babies and is usually a symptom of trouble in some other organ. In bottle-fed babies, diarrhoea and other intestinal disorders are more frequent.

During the first three months in particular it must be taken quite seriously and treated immediately. The danger of the complaint is that it causes rapid dehydration and loss of mineral salts. Dietary mistakes, but also overheating caused by too much bedding, specially during the summer, can cause diarrhoea.

The first measure is to cease giving milk, fat and sugar (this applies to diarrhoea in children of all ages). Small amounts of camomile tea or very weak ordinary tea are given, if necessary with a tiny amount of saccharine. During the first three months of life, babies must not be deprived of milk for more than two or three days, so if this is necessary, the doctor will prescribe a suitable alternative diet. A useful remedial recipe is carrot soup: Boil a pound of fresh carrots for at least two hours in a litre of water with a large pinch of salt. Strain, saving the water and topping up to bring back to one litre. Pass the carrots twice through a fine seive, then return the pulp to the water. Feed the baby with this mixture for five or more meals. If the baby is strong and over three months old, grated apple is also suitable: Grate a quarter of a good apple on a glass or plastic grater and feed with a spoon. Then grate the next quarter, and so on. This can also be given for five meals for at least two days during which all other food, even rusks, is strictly omitted. After the second day just over

1 oz. (30g) of the apple or carrot remedy is replaced by rice or oat gruel at each meal, after which there is a gradual transition back to normal food. At the earliest on the third day a dessertspoon of milk can be added to the meal. After this you may for some weeks have to resort to a patent baby food prescribed by the doctor.

Vomiting

Vomiting is in itself not an illness but rather an often rather dramatic symptom of an incipient or acute disorder.

There are, however, forms of vomiting caused by the nervous system. This is sudden and violent and indicates brain disease. Usually, however, vomiting is simply a sign of an upset stomach as a result of wrong feeding. The doctor will need to know whether the baby's tongue is clean or coated and whether there is diarrhoea as well as vomiting.

With ketotic vomiting the baby's mouth smells faintly of apples or acetone. This is a form of vomiting that can easily recur and must be treated by the doctor. He will prescribe enemas of sugar water, and perhaps ipecacuanha which is given orally drop by drop. If the child is given anything to drink he will immediately vomit again.

Pyloric spasm is another form of vomiting that occurs in very young babies. It is a cramp of the muscle at the exit of the stomach which prevents the food from passing into the intestines, causing it instead to be violently vomited. Babies with this complaint are hard to feed. Best of all is the mother's milk given by teaspoon. There are also good natural remedies, but if nothing helps, the doctor may have to send the baby to hospital. It is often possible to recognise babies with a tendency to this problem soon after birth by the tense expression on their faces, their nerviness and deep horizontal frowns on the forehead. I have noticed that babies whose mothers had been unable to come to terms with their pregnancy or who had been suffering from depression at the onset of pregnancy tend towards this complaint.

There are also children who have a virtuoso skill in the art of vomiting and use this ability to tyrannise their anxious parents. Babies and children also vomit if forced to eat more than they need. Older children also vomit out of fear of exams or other events at school or at home. Unsuitable medicaments, or actual poisons, also cause vomiting. And finally the nervous strain imposed by television watching has also now been recognised as a cause of vomiting.

Teething

Since the days of the ancient Greek physician Hippocrates there has been discussion of the symptoms of illness that occur in conjunction with the appearance of the first teeth. All mothers will have observed that before cutting a tooth the baby may refuse solid food, have diarrhoea, have a temperature of 101.3°F (38.5°C) or more, or show that their gums are tender by cramming their fists into their mouths, and of course crying. Some babies even start to cough, others suffer cramps, and when the eye-teeth come through they even sometimes contract conjunctivitis. The symptoms usually vanish as soon as the tooth is cut, and there is not a great deal that the doctor can do.

The cutting of the teeth, which are after all the hardest part of the whole organism, is a trial of strength for the whole human being. Vitamin B, especially B6, can sometimes help to alleviate teething symptoms.

There is a wide variety of timing in teething. In some families they come early, in others late. Rickets can cause exceptionally late teething, while some babies, for instance Napoleon, are born with teeth.

Usually children have 4 to 6 teeth by the beginning of their second year. As a rule of thumb we could say: In the sixth to ninth month the 2 middle lower incisors are cut; in the seventh to tenth month the 4 upper incisors; in the twelfth to fifteenth month the first upper molar on either side followed by the second pair of lower incisors, followed by the first lower molars; in the eighteenth to twenty-fourth month first the upper eye-teeth followed by the lower eye-teeth; in the thirtieth to thirty-sixth month finally the second pairs of molars appear, first the upper and then the lower.

Thus the milk teeth consist of 8 incisors, 8 molars and 4 eye-teeth, i.e. 20 teeth.

The second set of teeth, consisting usually of 32 teeth, starts to appear in the fifth or sixth year. It can be earlier or later but if it is much later the doctor should be consulted.

Usually a third pair of molars (top and bottom) appear. Then the milk teeth start to be pushed out, roughly in the order in which they came. Shortly before puberty the remaining canines appear, followed by the fourth pairs of molars (upper and lower), and finally, sometimes many years later, the fifth pairs of molars (wisdom teeth).

The beginning of the change of teeth shows that the child has reached a certain degree of maturity, both physically and psychologically. Thus as a general rule a child whose milk teeth have not even started to wobble should if possible not be sent to school. Of course the falling out of rotten teeth cannot be regarded as a sign of maturity. Usually it is a sign of a faulty diet, though some children are simply afflicted with bad teeth.

Regular care of the teeth should start at eighteen months. And even the milk teeth should be seen regularly by the dentist every six months.

Chills

Just as poison enters the organism via the mouth and stomach, so cold air can invade the organism through an exposed part of the skin, or through the mucous respiratory passages, the intestines, the bladder, the ears or eyes.

The result is a chill, which can afflict any part of the body, for instance as a cold in the nose, bronchitis, sinusitis, lumbago or flu. The ego is not working properly at the spot where the chill takes hold, and consequently disturbances arise in the organ which create favourable conditions for all sorts of agents that cause illness. These agents are thus not the primary cause but rather the consequence of the actual illness, but they bring about a worsening or spreading of the illness.

A useful remedy for a cold in the head region is a foot bath or even a full bath in which the heat of the water is gradually increased. (Footbaths with built in heater and thermostat are available on the market.) A sweat compress may also suffice (see page 197).

A herbal tea is a good additional remedy, for instance a mixture of equal amounts of peppermint, fennel and camomile, or great mullein, coltsfoot, icelandic moss and camomile with a large teaspoon of honey. The latter must be added to the tea when it is ready to drink but not hotter than 104°F (40°C), as otherwise the life forces of the honey are destroyed. These teas are sipped by the patient. Sytra Tea (Weleda) is good for a cough.

Another useful traditional remedy: Boil two large onions in ¾ of a litre of water for one hour, sieve and add honey as above. Give the patient 1 to 2 dessert-spoons every two hours.

For a more advanced cold or chill, a Schlenz Bath can be a great help (see page 200). Thus a great deal can be done to relieve colds and chills.

Abdominal pain and gastro-intestinal complaints

Children suffer abdominal pains for a variety of reasons, most of which are harmless. Some, however, must be taken seriously, so the doctor should be consulted if the pain lasts for more than an hour, especially if the child feels sick or actually does vomit. Take the child's temperature under the arm and in the rectum (each five minutes) and inform the doctor of both readings over the phone. (See page 189).

Sometimes the pains are caused by the food the child

eats, either because he has eaten too much or because the food is of poor quality or made unpalatable by chemical additives.

However, the possibility of appendicitis or something similar must always be borne in mind, since even small babies can have appendicitis, though this is more likely with babies fed on commercial baby foods. Children can also contract stomach ulcers, a consequence of the so-called 'civilised' foods of today with their predominance of sugar and white flour. Inflammation of the gall bladder and also jaundice are no longer rare, whereas forty years ago it was most unusual for a child to suffer from a liver or gall bladder complaint.

Usually abdominal pain, vomiting and diarrhoea are indications of poisoning or an intestinal problem, especially if the child has shivering fits, a headache and a dry or coated tongue.

With food poisoning usually all those who have eaten the contaminated dish are affected. But with gastroenteritis members of a family usually take it in turns to succumb. There is always a possibility of typhoid, especially in hot weather.

Small children usually complain of abdominal pain when they have a sore throat, especially in the early stages of the attack.

Newborn and small infants often suffer from wind and abdominal pain when breast-fed if the mother is too restless, anxious or agitated, or if she eats too much raw fruit, or drinks coffee or strong tea.

Abdominal cramps (colic) every few minutes interspersed with pain-free intervals followed by consti-

pation and vomiting point to the possibility of a twisting
of the intestines. This can occur in children as young as
four months. Either the intestine is blocked by twisting
into a loop, or the upper end of the intestines pushes
itself into the lower part. (I have seen a case where the
small intestine had passed right through the large
intestine and protruded for about 10 centimetres from
the rectum.) If such possibilities are borne in mind,
preventive measures can be taken before it is too late, so
consult the doctor in good time!

Children with poor appetites often have 'tummy
ache' before or during every meal from dread of the
daily torture of being forced to eat. It is quite wrong to
force unwilling children to eat, since this causes cramps
in stomach or intestines which make the digestive
glands cease the secretion of digestive juices, resulting
in actual inability to digest the unwelcome food.

Other children get tummy ache if they dread going to
school or are afflicted with other anxieties. Happy
excitement, for instance looking forward to a journey,
can also cause painful cramps in the digestive organs.
In fact excitement of all kinds can cause 'stomach
cramps', diarrhoea or vomiting.

Chemical medicaments, worm cures or laxatives can
cause intestinal allergies leading to painful irritation of
the intestinal mucous membranes. Fresh bread and
also vegetables, especially spinach, grown with artificial manure can all cause painful intestinal conditions.
Intestinal tuberculosis, which is very rare nowadays,
causes similar symptoms. Even grapes not properly
washed (first briefly in hot and then in cold water) and

other sprayed fruit eaten with its skin can cause serious symptoms.

The doctor should always be consulted, especially if the symptoms keep recurring, and if the mother knows the various possibilities she will be able to make valuable observations that can help the doctor in his diagnosis.

In obvious cases of cramp or colic, when there is no likelihood of appendicitis, relief can be obtained by applying a warmed bag of camomile flowers or hay-flowers (flores graminis) to the abdomen (See page 199).

Appendicitis

The danger with an inflammation of the appendix and the neighbouring intestine is that it might become perforated, allowing the contents of the intestine to spill into the abdominal cavity, causing peritonitis. Perforation can occur quite quickly, only a few hours after the onset of the abdominal pains, or it does not occur at all, which is usually the case.

Until quite recently every inflamed appendix was immediately removed, although in about eighty per cent of the cases the appendix itself was found to be not at all or only slightly inflamed. It was considered to be a superfluous organ that might have had some function during earlier phases of human evolution. Nowadays it has become apparent that it may not be as unimportant as had been thought but may have to do with the secretion of lymph active in increasing resistance to infections. I have rarely found it necessary to have an appendix operated. But diagnosis is very difficult as the symptoms are so varied. There may be virtually no pain, or no temperature. And when there is doubt, the patient should have the operation without delay. Even tiny babies can have acute inflammation of the appendix.

If a child suddenly stops playing and complains of tummy ache and feeling sick, he should be put to bed immediately. All inflammation needs peace and quiet and the child should be persuaded to lie as still as possible. If necessary his legs can be tied together with a scarf or nappy. After 20 minutes lying quietly the temperature can be taken (See *Taking the temperature*, page 189). Give absolutely *nothing* to eat or drink.

If the discomfort continues (sharp pains on the right side of the abdomen, first higher up and later lower down, feeling sick or vomiting, rapid pulse, an ailing demeanour and tense facial expression) the doctor should be called immediately, even in the middle of the night. Tell him the two temperature measurements (See page 190).

If the intestine is empty as a result of the child being given no food or drink, there is far less likelihood of perforation of the appendix. A small, gentle (balloon) enema can be given to clear the intestine, but on no account any laxative or laxative tea. The enema consists of no more than a little cool water. On no account should warm compresses be applied to the abdomen. The doctor will decide whether cold or other compresses should be applied.

If there is no need for an operation, which is usually

the case, medicinal treatment can be allowed to come into its own. There are anthroposophical and similar medicines and methods which can combat even acute appendicitis, and it is a serious mistake to believe that only antibiotics are suitable. This is also the case with peritonitis.

Orthodox medical methods have achieved a large increase in cures through the use of antibiotics. This is praiseworthy but was also highly necessary. Doctors using natural biological methods are anyway used to a high rate of success.

Pneumonia

A heavy cold, especially if it results from an attack of flu, can easily turn into pneumonia, particularly if a medicine has been given to suppress rather than loosen the cough. For instance with measles there is hardly likely to be a complication of pneumonia if the cough has not been suppressed with medicaments containing codeine.

Pneumonia may be recognised by the high temperature, the agitation of the child, the shallow breathing often accompanied by moaning, and the way the nostrils dilate every time a breath is exhaled. The child also has a very red face and often feels sharp pains in the chest. If the inflammation is just beginning, all these symptoms will be slight. The pain is not in the lungs but in the pleura or bronchial tubes.

In my experience, treatment with antibiotics is not necessary. I have always achieved perfect recovery without them. My aim is not to suppress the course of the illness but to help the patient while it runs its course. Without a doubt children who are helped through the illness in this way gain new and valuable capacities that help them to master life. If pneumonia is suspected, the doctor must be called immediately. He may prescribe compresses (See page 197).

Croup and diphtheria

Croup arises when there is a sudden swelling of the mucous membranes deep down in the throat and in the larynx, which can lead to a narrowing of the wind-pipe almost causing suffocation. The cough is dry and barking. The condition looks more alarming than it is, and if the mother keeps calm and does not excite the child, causing him to breathe irregularly, he will be able to get enough breath. So even if the first attack comes in the middle of the night and looks very alarming, keep calm! Try immediately to make the air in the bedroom as damp as possible, for instance by boiling an electric kettle. Or take the child into the bathroom and let hot water run into the bath, so that the child can breathe in the steam. Then put the child back to bed with the upper part of his body raised to ease his breathing.

Attacks of this kind usually occur at the beginning of winter or in February or March. They are without a temperature unless they are complicated by bronchitis or something similar. Usually the child will have been perfectly healthy during the day and then suddenly at about nine o'clock at night will be woken by the loud barking cough. The pattern will be repeated during the following evenings if the doctor has not succeeded in taking suitable measures. There are natural remedies which are very effective, and the doctor may also recommend hot compresses (See page 199). Children who have been overfed with milk or other foods are prone to these attacks of croup.

In contrast, diphtheria is dangerous, because the windpipe is coated with mucous. It is now very rare. The cough is a dry barking cough arising in the region of the larynx. It must not be confused with croup. Diphtheria is accompanied by a temperature, and a bad smell from the mouth. The doctor must verify the condition by an examination of the throat. The temperature with diphtheria is usually not more than 102.2°C (39°C), that is less than with flu or tonsillitis. The saliva and mucous expelled by the coughing are of course very infectious.

Inflammation of the middle ear

Inflammation of the middle ear can arise fairly easily as a complication of a bad cold or in particular of tonsillitis which has not been properly cured. With infants as well as older children it usually starts first at night with isolated sharp pain in the ear. The child wakes and cries. The following night the attacks are more frequent and the pain worse. Babies throw their head to and fro and rub the painful ear with their hand. There is also an acute form of the illness which sets in immediately with very bad pain.

The pain can often be soothed by pouring a few drops of warm milk or oil into the ear while pulling gently at the outer ear to help the liquid seep down to the ear drum while letting the air in the passage escape. (Method: Boil water and dip the bowl of a spoon into this to absorb the heat. Pour a few drops of sunflower, olive or Weleda silica oil into the spoon and wait for half a minute. The oil will then have the correct temperature for pouring into the ear.)

An onion poultice can help if the pain is very bad, as the onion draws the inflammation towards the outside (See page 204). But the doctor must be consulted.

Every domestic medicine chest should contain a paediatric analgesic for the relief of very bad pain.

If the child has a temperature, cold compresses on the calves can be applied to relieve the pressure of blood in the head, though not to completely dampen down the temperature. A sweat compress or Schlenz Bath is very important on the morning after a night of earache. In addition the doctor will prescribe one of the biological remedies that has proved successful with ear inflammation.

Lancing of the ear drum is only necessary in rare cases. If the ear drum bursts of its own accord, careful rinsing with camomile will assist the discharge of pus. See that the child lies on the sick ear to allow the rinse to drain away. The child will have to remain under the care of the doctor to ensure that the condition does not become chronic. If the condition worsens to the extent of a mastoid infection, even this can be cured in most cases by medical treatment. If this fails, there will have to be an operation to prevent the pus from making its way into the blood vessels of the brain.

Acute tonsillitis

The doctor must always be consulted when the tonsils are inflamed, since there are many forms of tonsillitis. The mother, for instance cannot distinguish between tonsillitis and diphtheria, and though the latter is a 'dying' disease its pattern of recurrence is not known and one cannot be too careful. There are also other malignant forms of tonsillitis which may at first appear quite harmless.

The mother can support the work of the doctor by giving the child as little protein as possible, i.e. no meat or eggs, while giving instead fresh lemon, orange and raw vegetable juices. The digestion may need to be supported with a milk laxative or a laxative tea. Very small children can be given an enema.

Serious illness can often be averted by giving the child as soon as possible an intensive footbath (Schlenz Footbath, see page 200). For a throat compress, lemon is suitable. Make incisions all round half an unsprayed lemon under water in a bowl, then press the lemon against the bottom of the bowl, thus squeezing out the juice. (Half a lemon is sufficient for one compress.) If the lemon is sprayed, just squeeze the juice into the water without immersing the skin. If the nose is blocked, let the child inhale the steam from camomile tea.

An effective preventive measure: For about six weeks during the autumn wash the child's neck and upper trunk with sea-salt water daily.

Vaccination — Fundamental considerations

What is vaccination? In general, vaccination is carried out as a protection against certain infectious diseases. Infection is caused by the invasion of the organism by bacteria or viruses (or innumerable other agents or toxic substances) leading to the typical symptoms of the illness in question. Some examples are: pneumonia, pyelonephritis, typhoid fever, dysentery, lung tuberculosis, polio, venereal diseases, and also the diseases of childhood discussed in this book.

A number of these illnesses, e.g. the childhood diseases, polio, tuberculosis, and (if the patient survives) smallpox and tetanus only attack an individual once. After the attack he is immune.

The explanation for this is that during an illness of this kind certain antibodies form in the blood of the afflicted person and annihilate the cause of the illness. These antibodies remain in the blood throughout life, preventing a new infection with the illness even if the person is in contact with others who are infected. The time it takes for the antibodies to form is called the immunisation phase.

Other infectious illnesses such as pneumonia or flu do not result in permanent immunisation. The antibodies disappear again after a while and the person can be infected anew.

A new step was taken when medical science learnt how to bring about immunisation artificially. Jenner and Koch were pioneers in this. A weakened form of the cause of the disease was inoculated under the skin, thus causing a controlled infection.

Unfortunately the hopes raised by this new method have not been entirely fulfilled. This will be discussed in more detail.

First, however, let us mention briefly so-called passive vaccination. In this case, serum from the blood of animals containing the immunisation substance is injected. This method is usually used where rapid protection is required. The best-known of these is the anti-tetanus serum for injuries. In a similar way, though completely naturally, breast-fed babies are protected during their early months because they imbibe antibodies with their mother's milk.

When a baby is subjected to active immunisation, a powerful biological revolution takes place from which he takes a long time to recover. All the greater is the strain resulting from multiple vaccination. Threefold, fourfold and even fivefold vaccinations force me to conclude that the infant organism is regarded as an automaton into which any number of antigens can be introduced which then lead to the same number of immunities. This is an invasion of medicine by a computer mentality.

It was high time to oppose this dangerous enthusiasm for vaccination, especially with vaccines (such as the fivefold vaccine) which have been insufficiently tested. Recently a child died two days after being treated with the fivefold vaccine. Also the assertion* that the first vaccination against smallpox should take

---

* In a number of countries, including Britain, routine vaccination of small children against smallpox is no longer undertaken.

place during the early months of life strikes me as being highly doubtful, especially as a considerable amount has been published asserting that this method is of little value. In recent years, more people have died in England from smallpox vaccination than from smallpox. For smallpox vaccination I strongly advise the new dry vaccine.

Over the years it has become evident that the attitude to vaccination represented in this book coincides with that of many specialists in the field. Professor Stickel, Director of the Munich Institute for Vaccination, for instance, warns against misuse and excessive use of vaccination. He suggests that smallpox vaccination, obviously only given to healthy children, should not be administered before the second year. 'Problem children', that is any child whose physical or psychological development is not normal, must not be vaccinated. No vaccination for measles. No multiple vaccinations. Tetanus vaccination not until the second or third year. And in general, vaccination should only be undertaken if it is really necessary.

Gynaecologists, furthermore, state that smallpox vaccination should be avoided throughout pregnancy, because of the danger to the child. Small children should also not be vaccinated if their mother is pregnant again.

The fact that, despite all this, the vaccination of babies and infants persists, comes about because they show very little reaction, whereas older children can react with cramps, fever, vomiting and confusion. It is now known that small children react so mildly because they do not yet possess sufficient strength with which to counteract the vaccination. Thus the danger is all the greater that the vaccine will affect the brain. In the embryo, the skin and the membranes of the brain develop from the same germ cell. Thus all vaccinations applied in or under the skin (smallpox, tuberculosis, whooping cough, measles, etc.) can easily affect the brain.

A further risk is presented by multiple vaccinations or by single vaccinations administered at short intervals: After a vaccination, during the immunisation phase (see above), the patient is busy reacting to one particular vaccination and is therefore not able to react to others. (See below.)

It is most essential to realise, furthermore, that immunity does not last a lifetime, whereas an attack of a childhood disease in the natural way does lead to life-long immunity. In most cases protection through vaccination lasts only for a few years. Hence the many repeat vaccinations that are necessary, for instance for smallpox, measles, polio etc. And hence also the danger of the child contracting the disease despite the vaccination. When this happens the illness is usually particularly serious and dangerous. These children obviously have little capacity to react out of themselves.

It is obvious that the vaccination question requires a great deal of responsible consideration. Every case is different and must be considered individually. All fanatical advertising in favour of vaccination should be condemned, especially as it usually engenders excessive fear.

In the United States, where there has for years been no case of smallpox but where there have been numerous cases of damage from vaccination, the abolition of smallpox vaccination is being considered. Similarly in Japan. In the Federal Republic of Germany, smallpox vaccination is no longer compulsory (since 1976), except in certain cases: re-vaccination of twelve-year-olds who were vaccinated as small children, for certain professions, and if there is a danger of infection. It is felt by the authorities that the abolition of compulsion is justified on the ground of the success of the World Health Organisation's programme to eradicate the disease. This sensible decision has furthermore surely come about as a result of the realisation that the advantages have been exaggerated in relation to the tragic damage (and the resulting costs) that can ensue.

Epidemics are as unpredictable as the weather; our knowledge of their laws is full of gaps. It seems to me that we should not rely too much on statistics nor place too much confidence in vaccination alone.

Since the introduction of oral vaccination the incidence of polio has dwindled to a few isolated cases; certainly cases of paralysis and death hardly occur any more. However, I venture to doubt whether the prevention of paralysis really means that the polio problem can be regarded as overcome. Diphtheria is an equally dangerous illness which has at present become rare. Yet nobody can seriously maintain that the relatively small proportion of diphtheria vaccinations is the cause of this reduction; in fact the disease began to dwindle before the diphtheria serum was even invented. Epi-

demics of plague, cholera, typhus and spotted fever
have 'disappeared' from the civilised world without any
vaccination, perhaps because of improved hygienic
conditions. But is this the only explanation? In my
opinion there are other aspects to consider with regard
to illness and epidemics in addition to the fact that they
are caused by bacteria or viruses.

The four parts of the human being, physical body, life
forces, soul forces and spiritual forces have been
mentioned a number of times in this book. I would like
to maintain that when these four members are in
harmony, infections are warded off or overcome. Only
when they are in disharmony can infections take hold.
This applies even more to the virus infections which
threaten us today than to the bacterial epidemics of the
past. It must be admitted that the pressures of life today
lead to considerable disturbances of the interplay
between man's four members and from this point of
view it would seem that there is no lack of opportunity
for virus infections to take hold.

Vaccination, however, is not the only protection.
Professor Pette, a well-known vaccination expert and
neurologist, wrote a few years ago: 'Every vaccination is
a serious interference with the human organism.' This
throws light on the fact that the general standard of
health in countries which undertake a great deal of
vaccination is considerably lower than in countries
which have approached vaccination with more hesitation. Of course there are also other causes for this
phenomenon, but it nevertheless gives cause for
concern.

Even if it turns out in the end that vaccination does give proper protection to the individual, there are a number of grave objections to its use. In some countries infants receive as many as fourteen injections in the first three months of life and the number is likely to increase as new vaccines are discovered. Doctors who include all four aspects of the human being in their considerations cannot but be exceedingly worried by this prospect. It seems extremely likely that the general resistance to illness of those vaccinated will decrease progressively, that their ability to stand up to stress will decrease, and that sterility, allergies and above all liver damage will result from increased vaccination. This is already becoming apparent in the poor health standards of those countries with the most comprehensive vaccination programmes.

Another serious objection to vaccination is that it obscures the real reasons for the increasing incidence of new virus infections. Since reforms are always unpopular, we shall no doubt continue to live unhealthy lives, making light of malnutrition arising from poor food quality, persisting in overstimulating our nervous systems, and turning to the panacea of the latest vaccine whenever we need it.

The illusion that we can drag from the earth unlimited supplies of food if only we put back enough mineral fertilisers and kill enough pests with chemical sprays seems to me similar to the illusion that we can continue indefinitely to combat illness with vaccination.

However, I must stress that I do not want to prevent

anyone from having himself or his children vaccinated. Particularly with polio it has been shown that fear increases the chances of contracting the disease. It cannot be my business to prevent anyone from accepting vaccination. So far, for instance, oral vaccination against polio seems to be a complete success. Nevertheless, this was also thought to be the case with smallpox vaccination until experience laid the foundation for doubts. So let us not rely too heavily on vaccination, which may turn out to be an illusion based on wishful thinking. Instead let us do all we can to increase the body's natural resistance to epidemics. There are plenty of suggestions in this book.

Frequent questions about vaccination
- *In the case of oral vaccination against polio is there any danger of the virus being transferred to unvaccinated persons?*

Experience has shown that the amount of virus which may pass from treated to untreated persons is not enough to cause an infection. It is conceivable that in the case of a small child receiving this vaccination, others in the same household might be infected but so far this has not been known to happen. Of course extra cleanliness must be observed, especially in dealing with the nappy or potty of the child.

- *Who may definitely not be vaccinated?*

Anyone suffering from an acute illness with or without fever; anyone with a stomach or intestinal complaint (diarrhoea, gastritis, enteritis, etc.); anyone undergoing a course of treatment with cortisone;

anyone with one of the infectious children's diseases. For smallpox vaccination the patient's skin must in addition be absolutely healthy. For vaccination in pregnancy see below.

- *How much time must elapse between vaccinations?*

After a first vaccination against smallpox, and after subsequent vaccinations if pustules have appeared, at least six weeks must elapse before other vaccinations are undertaken. If in the case of second or subsequent vaccinations only a small lump appears, other vaccinations can be undertaken after a week.

After BCG vaccination against tuberculosis at least three months must elapse before a first smallpox vaccination is undertaken. After oral vaccination against polio and after yellow fever vaccination four weeks must elapse before a smallpox vaccination is undertaken. A three week gap is sufficient after other vaccinations.

If tetanus serum or other animal serum (horse, cow or sheep) has been injected, three weeks must elapse before smallpox vaccination is undertaken.

Vaccination during pregnancy

In the first three months all vaccination must be avoided, especially polio and smallpox. If at all possible it should be avoided during the whole of pregnancy, even if needed for foreign travel.

The virus in smallpox vaccination can pass from the blood of the expectant mother to that of the baby. This is all the more reason to avoid it during pregnancy, especially in the first three and in the final months. For the same reason oral vaccination with live virus against polio should be avoided, especially during the early months. Treatment with BCG vaccine against tuberculosis is only recommended if the expectant mother has unavoidable close contact with a patient suffering from open tuberculosis where isolation is impossible.

Important note on vaccination

For every vaccination give the person Weleda Thuja D30 drops starting on the day of the vaccination (3-5 drops morning and evening on an empty stomach). For smallpox vaccination continue till the pustules have disappeared.

Fever resulting from vaccination can lead to brain damage and the use of Thuja D30 with every vaccination helps protect the brain.

3. CHILDHOOD ILLNESSES

Incubation periods and duration of infectiousness

	Incubation period	Duration of infectiousness
Diphtheria	2-7 days	Patient is no longer infectious after the third negative throat and nose swab
Whooping cough	8-21 days	When the whooping stops

Measles	9-11 days	After three weeks
Polio*	8-14 days	Isolation usually 6 weeks
Mumps	16-22 days	Patient is no longer infectious when all symptoms have disappeared
Scarlet fever	1-7 days	Isolation usually 6 weeks
Chicken pox	2-3 weeks	Patient no longer infectious after 3 weeks
German measles	2-3 weeks	Patient no longer infectious after 10 days

* Polio and some virus diseases are only infectious in exceptional circumstances.

Measles

With the childhood illnesses which share the symptom of a red rash (measles, scarlet fever, German measles) the purpose of the illness is particularly clear.

Most children need measles for their healthy development and are thus 'inwardly prepared' for the illness. This is why they nearly always catch the disease if they contact infection. It is quite an exception not to have gone through measles. Even brief contact with a patient in the infectious stage, especially in the days before the rash appears, will lead in 10 or 11 days to the onset of the initial catarrh, followed in three or four days by the outbreak of the rash. The picture painted by the rash on the child's skin reveals the nature of this illness. As the temperature rises, the facial skin swells, making the features indistinct. The mucous membranes of the eyes, nose, throat, larynx and windpipe are also swollen and inflamed and show a liquid discharge. Starting behind the ears a patchy red rash spreads over the head and then over the whole body as well as the internal mucous membranes. The child develops conjunctivitis, avoids the light, and has a cold in the nose and catarrh in the respiratory passages. Not infrequently the pressure on the brain increases, with consequent cramps or disturbances of consciousness. The white spots which appear inside the cheeks identify measles finally, since it is not often easy to distinguish the rash from that of German measles.

After three of four days the rash fades, the facial swelling recedes, the inflammation of the mucous membranes diminishes, the cough and cold cease, and the child recovers rapidly. There are, however, cases in which the cough is very bad and persistent and the child feels very ill for quite some time.

The following remarks may help in the treatment and nursing of measles: All unnecessary treatment should be avoided. In particular the temperature should not be suppressed, even if it exceeds 104°F (40°C). Similarly the cough must not be suppressed. Such measures can lead to the justifiably dreaded pneumonia arising as a complication of measles. The inflamed state of the mucous membranes leads unavoidably to considerable coughing. Weleda Cough Elixir is a good loosener and brings relief. Nothing much more need be done, as the

cough will diminish after two or three days anyway. No
chest compresses should be applied while the rash is
visible. If the child is very restless he can be given a
quick wipe with vinegar water. To avoid cooling off,
work quickly and rub energetically all over the trunk
and legs with a mixture of two thirds luke warm water
and one third wine or cider vinegar. Do not dry. If the
child avoids the light the room should be darkened. The
bowel must be moved daily, if necessary with the help of
an enema. The diet should consist above all of fruit juice
and fresh fruit, or with small children hot milk diluted
half and half with mineral water. No protein-rich so-
called 'nourishing' food should be given and the return
to a normal diet should not start till the child demands
it. The child must stay in bed for ten days and have a
further ten to fourteen days quiet at home. When the
fever has abated, Weleda Waldon II is a good tonic, but
so are a number of natural calcium preparations with
additional iron.

Scarlet fever

Scarlet fever is much more uncommon than measles,
and serious cases are now rare. In contrast to measles,
though, even light cases of scarlet fever must be taken
seriously, especially the 'second phase' of the illness,
which usually commences during the third week, since
there is a danger of complications involving the kidneys or ears. Scarlet fever is far less infectious than
measles, but the contagion is erratic, so strict isolation is
necessary for six weeks.

The illness usually starts suddenly without much

preliminary discomfort. The initial symptoms are high temperature, vomiting, headache, and in small children sometimes convulsions. Soon the tonsils become inflamed and the soft palate turns a flaming red. The itchy rash appears on the very first day, on the neck and then spreading over the whole torso. The thickly clustered minute red spots gradually merge to make a uniform redness of the skin. Quite often, however, the rash hardly develops and can only be detected by careful scrutiny of the groin and the inside of the thighs. Thus it is frequently overlooked. Diagnosis is helped by the strawberry tongue which appears after three or four days. After about five days, the skin redness gradually fades. In the second or third week the outer skin begins to peel, first in small flakes but later often in large shreds. There are a number of feverish illnesses that are accompanied by rashes that resemble that of scarlet fever. In some cases final diagnosis is only possible when the skin starts to peel.

The doctor must definitely be consulted when the child has scarlet fever, but the modern rapid cure with antibiotics should be avoided if at all possible.

During the first five or six days the child is given only fruit juice or raw fruit, until the tongue is clean again. Daily bowel movement is assured with the help of Weleda Clairo Tea or if necessary with an enema. If the constipation is very solid, a camomile enema can be given. The child must be kept strictly in bed even in the third week, since this is the point when the ears or kidneys can become affected.

Chicken pox

Chicken pox is extremely infectious. The child does not have a very high temperature. The rash consists of tiny watery blisters covering the whole body, including the scalp, the inside of the mouth and the mucous membranes of eyes, ears and genitals. They last for about five days, during which some heal while new ones continue to appear. Sometimes the patient has only a few of these blisters, while in other epidemics the body is covered with hundreds of them. The rash is extremely irritating, and if it is extensive the child must be kept in bed for a few days. If scratched, the blisters will leave small scars. To relieve the itching, dab the places with vinegar water ($2/3$ water, $1/3$ vinegar) and afterwards sprinkle with powder.

German measles

This is such a mild illness that it hardly needs any treatment, except perhaps the many lymph gland swellings, particularly on the back of the neck. Strict isolation is unnecessary, and the child can return to school after 10 days. Lifelong immunity is assured. The rash sometimes resembles a light attack of measles, at others it is more like that of scarlet fever. (Regarding German measles in pregnancy, see page 29).

Mumps

Mumps is a virus infection. Infection usually takes place from person to person, more rarely via healthy carriers, and most rarely via infected objects. It is a very infectious disease, except that small babies do not so easily catch it. It is rare for a person to have the illness more than once. In recent years it has become more serious than it used to be.

The temperature is usually high for a short time. The parotid salivary gland in the neck swells, often on one side at a time, and is painful when pressed. Chewing is painful, and the ear can hurt. Sometimes the submandibular salivary gland is also affected. Complications can be inflammation of the scrotum and also meningitis, but this is unusual before puberty.

Treatment should not be taken lightly. If the child has a temperature he should be kept in bed, preferably for too long rather than too short a time. Let him rinse his mouth and gargle with sage tea or Weleda Mouth Wash and make sure his bowel movements are adequate. The swollen glands may be covered with cotton wool soaked in hot oil or with an ointment prescribed by the doctor. The diet should be vegetarian with plenty of fruit and as little protein as possible.

Whooping cough

Many doctors still regard this illness as a threat to the life of babies and small children. Certainly in the past thousands of children did die of it every year and deaths do still occur occasionally.

More than with any other illness it is now possible to vouch statistically for the efficacy of the superior therapeutic effectiveness of natural remedies and methods. Treated in this way, no otherwise healthy child, or even small baby, dies of whooping cough today. The complications of this illness, which usually involve the brain, are also avoided with these methods.

The main innovation is that the whooping attacks are not suppressed but rather helped to take place, while the cramp is loosened to the extent of no longer being dangerous.

Preventive vaccination should be avoided, for whooping cough is most certainly a 'healthy disease'.

Of course this is not to say that the mother will not have a good many disturbed nights. But the attacks look worse than they are, which becomes obvious when you see the child resume playing happily as soon as the attack is over. Sensible parents will come to terms with even the heavy attacks, which occur for a duration of 8 to 10 days, when they understand that this is a crisis which will have a favourable outcome. (Lighter attacks may go on for much longer.) If the parents overcome their worries, the atmosphere in the house will be free from anxiety. When the child has an attack, encourage him not to worry and let him spit out the catarrh or even vomit his recent meal. After the attack, first give the child his medicine and then a small snack. Thus food is not taken at the normal mealtimes but little by little after each attack. It should be light, in small portions and without crumbs which might unnecessarily stimulate a new attack of coughing. Children who do not eat much usually pass through the coughing phase particularly rapidly. Some loss of weight is of no account, since the child's subsequent excellent appetite will soon put this right.

The medicament that has achieved the success described above is Pertudoron I and II (Weleda). The doctor will advise about the dosage, but do not give it too frequently.

The course of the illness can be complicated by bronchitis or some other acute attacks.

Apart from the light and sparse diet, the mother can also help the child considerably by remaining absolutely calm. The room may be aired after each attack. While the attacks are at their most violent, there is no point in taking the child out into the open air. Rapid movements bring on attacks. Cold wind, especially east wind, is particularly unsuitable. Relief can also be given with hot chest poultices or compresses with warm beeswax for ten minutes (See page 203). It is superfluous to travel with the child for the sake of a change of air. It unnecessarily spreads the infection to other children and a change of air can sometimes make the attacks worse. In some cases a flight lasting an hour during which an altitude of 3000 metres is maintained for at least 20 minutes can help to alleviate attacks. But this can frighten the child, which is of course counterproductive.

Parents and especially grandparents can catch whooping cough from the children. Adults will suffer from a persistent, violent cough, especially in the morning. Pertudoron is of great help to adults too, and they should start to take it at the first sign, though not more frequently than at two-hour intervals, taking the drops alternately. The number of drops according to the age of the patient.

Polio

As a result of the widespread use of oral vaccination against polio, this disease is at the moment on the wane. But to assist an early diagnosis, should it occur, the following description is included.

The illness usually starts with a feverish attack of one kind or another (a cold, flu, bronchitis, acute diarrhoea, middle ear infection, tonsillitis, etc.). Then the temperature goes down for one or several days, after which it rises again. This is accompanied by bad headaches and pain in the spine, particularly in the loins, spreading into the abdomen and thighs. Nearly always there is also pain and stiffness in the neck. The doctor must be consulted immediately. (For the treatment of polio, see Zur Linden *Geburt und Kindheit,* Vittorio Klostermann Verlag, Frankfurt.)

4. CHRONIC ILLNESSES

Hearing defects

If a child shows no reactions to noise in his second year, or if he has shown no signs of starting to speak by the time he is eighteen months old, hearing problems must be suspected.

During the past twenty years the number of children with hearing problems seems to have increased. This may be connected with the increase of loud noise in our environment. Deafness can also follow from chicken pox.

However, much progress has also been made in the treatment even of severe deafness in children. The earlier the problem is discovered the better. Hearing aids can now utilise even the smallest remnants of hearing ability, thus making it possible for even severely deaf children to learn to speak.

Children with deafness in the family should be examined as early as possible, certainly long before they go to school.

Sight defects

Normally the proper functioning of the eyes is not achieved till the fourth or fifth year. The child only learns gradually to understand the sight impressions he receives daily from the moment of birth. Thus it is quite normal for a one-year old to look at a picture book upside down, to miss an object he is reaching for, or to try to touch the moon. On the other hand there is a great danger that sight disturbances (for instance short or long sight, colour blindness, or even congenital blindness) are overlooked or discovered too late. In families who suffer from these problems they are more likely to be noticed.

Anything unusual should be reported to the doctor, for instance lack of expression, either of joy or sorrow, in the eyes, or lack of reaction in the pupils. These decrease in bright light or on looking into the distance and increase in poor light or when the eyes are closed; other stimuli, such as pain or noise, cause the pupils to change as well. Large pupils can be a sign of short sightedness and small pupils of long sightedness. There may also be unusual movements of the eyeballs, such as trembling or twitching.

Congential squinting is more common. It can be caused by disturbances in the balance of the eye muscles or by paralysis of some of those muscles. Medical treatment is necessary.

Since the child grasps his surroundings in the first place through his eyes, it is most important to make sure that he is seeing a clear and not a clouded picture (long or short sight), and a single rather than a double image (squinting). It is obvious that someone seeing a distorted world will be a prey to psychological disturbances and be unable to think clearly.

There are many ways in which the doctor can help in these problems, starting with spectacles, which need not be a cause for distress.

Jaw deformation (and prevention)

When the teeth start to appear, it is frequently found that bottom and top teeth do not meet properly. If the child sucks his thumb, this condition is made worse. Usually the position adopted by the hand is such that the upper jaw is pushed forwards and the lower backwards. If incisors have already appeared, the upper ones are pushed outwards while the lower ones cannot grow upwards properly. The bottom lip then usually inserts itself between the upper and lower front teeth thus making the situation even worse, so that the child can only bring his lips together with an effort. Air breathed in through the nose is cleaned, warmed, humidified and to a great extent made germ-free. None of this happens when the child breathes through his mouth. In addition, he will tend to swallow air and there will be disturbances and congestion in the blood and lymph circulations of the throat. Faulty positioning and functioning of the mouth and all its parts, combined with faulty breathing, leads to functional, digestive and metabolic disturbances.

Special dummies (NUK-Sauger dummies in West Germany) can help prevent these deformations.

But once the jaw is deformed, many years of patient treatment are needed before the situation can be corrected. The best time to start correction is at the change of teeth.

Faulty posture and spinal curvature

Spinal curvature or faulty posture with the resulting damage this can do is often the result of early forced sitting and standing. A child with this problem has a hollow chest, the spine curves backwards at the top and correspondingly forwards in the small of the back tilting the pelvis forward and pushing the abdomen forward. The head is bent forwards and the shoulders are rounded. The legs are knock-kneed and the feet flat. The child will need orthopaedic help, and very good results are also achieved with curative eurythmy.

Anaemia

Anaemia usually arises through an iron deficiency in the blood and can occur in the first few weeks of life. Those particularly susceptible are the children of anaemic mothers, premature babies, babies who are born well after the expected date, and also twins. The signs are pallor, apathy, tiredness and lack of appetite.

The child is also susceptible to any infections in the neighbourhood and usually has poor posture.

He will require medical treatment and also dietary help, as well as a great deal of sun and fresh air.

Nettle rash

Nettle rash and similar allergic reactions will continue to increase the more we add chemical substances to our food, our clothes, our washing and cleaning materials, and the more we indulge in vaccinations of all kinds.

In some cases it is also an allergy against certain foods, e.g. strawberries, fish, seafood, or even milk when it touches the skin, that can cause similar eruptions to appear within seconds.

There are a number of preparations the doctor can prescribe for nettle rash. In addition to these, make sure that the child's bowel and bladder are emptied, and give fresh fruit and vegetable juice without sugar, as little protein as possible, no white sugar or chocolate or cocoa, very little salt. The itchy parts can be treated with vinegar water ($2/3$ water and $1/3$ wine or cider vinegar), or powder. If the itching persists, give pure cod-liver oil ($1/2$ to 1 dessertspoon twice daily). Compresses or baths with Weleda Lavender Bath Lotion (Weleda), or Aesculus Essence (Wala) also help sooth itching.

Eczema

There are as many reasons for eczema as there are reasons for the organism to react with a skin rash or eczema. This can take numerous forms, for instance red patches of various kinds, lumps, small blisters, scales or scabs. In most cases the cause is an allergy.

It is for the doctor to determine the cause, and the mother should not treat the rash herself with creams or ointments, particularly those containing coaltar or cortisone. Often the liver or spleen are not in order in an eczema sufferer. But disturbances in other organs can also cause skin trouble. Treatment with medicines should always be accompanied by external treatment. Often dietary change will be required. White sugar can cause itching. For some eczemas, milk will have to be avoided (see page 108).

In very persistent cases, the ability of the metabolism to react can be stimulated by a course of 10 to 12 fever-producing baths. This is for instance the case with psoriasis.

As a general rule it can be said that weeping rashes should be treated with damp compresses or baths, for instance with Aesculus Essence and definitely not with greasy ointments. When the irritation has improved, oil or ointments may be useful.

Enlarged tonsils and adenoids

If acute tonsillitis (see page 160), which can occur as early as the first year, is not carefully treated medically until the tonsil swelling has completely subsided, this can be the start of an affliction with enlarged tonsils and/or adenoids which can plague the whole of childhood. The general health of the child can suffer considerably under this strain. It is not sufficiently realised that swollen tonsils and adenoids also block all the passages of the nose, preventing these from being used properly in breathing.

There are a number of natural remedies that can help in treating both acute and chronic tonsillitis. But even with these there are a certain number of failures which have to be treated surgically.

Children who have a tendency towards these inflammations should be taken for their holidays to the mountains or to the seaside. Delicate children will need the warmer resorts, while any coast will suit stronger children.

Chapter Twelve

NURSING

It is hoped that the following descriptions of a number of nursing procedures will help the mother to assist the doctor. She should work with him and not on her own without consultation.

Many of these practical nursing traditions are fast disappearing and perhaps these descriptions will help save them from being forgotten forever.

They help the parents to work preventively against illnesses, to alleviate the sick child's distressing symptoms, and to create and maintain a healthy basis for life.

The unrestrained taking of tablets and pills should be seen for what it is, so that people may return to placing their confidence in the healing forces of nature and to an understanding of natural methods of healing.

The mother's love

A baby's healthy development depends to a far higher degree than most mothers realise on the daily intimate contact between mother and child. Far from love being 'just' a feeling and nothing concrete, the way a child thrives proves that though love may not be visible its effects are recognisable and perceptible.

Babies in hospital are prone to infection just because, despite even the greatest devotion on the part of the nurses, the mother's love is lacking.

Though the physical link with the mother is severed at birth, this is only the very first necessary step on the way to independent existence. The baby still needs the mother's physical proximity as she picks him up in her arms and places him beside her in bed. This encloses him ever and again in her motherly warmth so that he is totally surrounded by her ambience. Only the mother completely and utterly understands her child's needs which are at first almost wholly physical but soon become psychological as well.

Children who are separated from their mother during their first year, for whatever reason, suffer damage without any doubt, and only the most devoted care by other people can hope to compensate for this to some degree. Every unnecessary absence of the mother should therefore be avoided. Some forms of schizophrenia can now be attributed in decisive measure to disturbances of the links between mother and child in early infancy.

Mothers who go out to work should do so in the knowledge that they are definitely harming their children, even if they seem to thrive for the moment. Not until they are three years old are children independent enough to cope with their mother's absence.

Behaviour and facial expression of the sick child

When a child falls sick suddenly, it is useful for the doctor if the mother can describe his behaviour and expression when she telephones him or as soon as he arrives.

The way the child shows he is in pain is particularly revealing. It is difficult to glean anything from the baby's face, since if he is screaming it will be bright red, while his mouth will be wide open and his eyes screwed shut. He is likely to howl with abandon regardless of whether the pain is in his tummy, head, ears or even just the mucous membranes in his mouth as a result of teething. If the pain is due to teething, he will be trying to stuff his little fist into his mouth. Abdominal pain (colic) will make him draw up his legs suddenly and then push away again with his feet, and his tummy will be as hard as a board. Thus his limbs show us where the pain is situated. Earache will make him throw his head to and fro while he clumsily tries to stroke the painful ear. If he is crying because of pneumonia, which can be very painful owing to the accompanying pleurisy, his mouth will hardly be open but his eyes will be wide open and shiny with fever. His eyebrows will be drawn up in a frown and his mouth turned down at the corners. The pain in the pleura will force him to dampen the actual screaming. The characteristic breathing is the most important sign of pneumonia, since the doctor can often not hear anything through his stethoscope while the illness is still confined to the inner recesses of the lungs. From time to time, or constantly, the child breathes out in an audible sigh while the nostrils open wide. Peritonitis causes quick, shallow breathing interspersed with an occasional deep sighing exhalation. A child with meningitis wears a determined, thoughtful, rather fixed serious expression. His eyes will be sensitive to light, which in turn leads to a vertical frown on the brow. His glance is absent and his mouth firmly shut except when he occasionally emits a piercing scream. The limbs are usually still. A small child with pyelonephritis usually makes small agitated movements with his trunk, hollowing or even arching his back, and also makes strange twisting movements with his hands, of which the palms are burning hot.

Mention has already been made of the characteristic sleep position of the healthy child, with his arms raised one on either side of his head, and of the sick child whose arms lie at his sides. Remember also that the delicate perfume of small babies fades at the onset of an illness.

Observation of the child's behaviour continues to be most important for the doctor well beyond infancy, since most two or three-year-olds are still unable to give useful information as to 'where it hurts'. Some children who have had uncomfortable experiences with the doctor will also try to dissemble in order to avoid examination or another bout of treatment.

The doctor's diagnosis is also helped by observing the type of cough (dry, cramped, moist, sighing, hollow or whooping) or the type and consistency of vomiting (spluttering, pouring, with slime or the contents of the stomach, or with blood or consisting entirely of blood), as well as urine and faeces. Samples of excretions from bladder, bowel, vagina, nose or ears should be preserved for the doctor.

Taking the temperature
Ascertaining the exact temperature is very important and with small children taking the temperature in the rectum is the most reliable method, though if the child struggles this is virtually impossible. However, if he has

been used to this method from infancy he will not be afraid and there is absolutely no need for the method to be painful. Hold the well greased thermometer lightly between thumb and forefinger and insert into the rectum. It is best for a small baby to lie on his back while you hold his feet up with your free hand. Older children can lie on their side or tummy.

Older children can have their temperature taken in the mouth (under the tongue). Taking the temperature under the arm is not suitable with children as they cannot grip the thermometer tightly enough. Sometimes the temperature can be taken in the groin. The mercury should be well shaken down and the thermometer is kept in place for at least five minutes.

If appendicitis is suspected, take the temperature under the arm first, making sure that the child grips the thermometer tightly. Then take the temperature again in the rectum. The normal difference between external and internal temperature is 0.35°F (0.5°C). If the internal temperature is more than 0.35°F above the external measurement, an abdominal inflammation can be suspected. The doctor should be called, even at night, and told of the difference between the measurements.

There is no point taking the temperature within two hours after a meal, as digestion usually causes the temperature to rise. The best times are in the morning when the child wakes and in the afternoon between 3.30 and 4.30. (See also *The healing power of fever*, p.131)

Diet during acute illness

The main rule as regards diet in any acute illness, whether feverish or not, is to give little food. Feed the child only if he wants something and do not give so-called 'nourishing food', i.e. meat, broth or eggs. It is better to go hungry, because the digestive juices in mouth, stomach and intestines are greatly reduced or even absent in acute illness. Food is therefore not properly digested and only causes discomfort. All the child's forces are needed to combat the illness and it is not serious if some weight is lost, since most of this is fluid, which is easily lost when the child is ill or has a temperature but is just as easily restored afterwards, especially if the child's appetite has not been spoiled for months ahead by having been forced to eat.

It is best to offer small amounts of fresh fruit juices and fresh fruit, e.g. oranges, apples, berries or whatever is in season. Take care to peel sprayed fruits!

If the stomach is not affected by the illness and there is no vomiting or diarrhoea, the child can have warm milk. It is best to remove the cream and dilute the milk with herb tea or mineral water since this makes it more digestible. Grain coffee with a little honey can also be recommended. If the doctor does not specify, give very weak ordinary tea or preferably camomile, peppermint, rose hip or yarrow tea. Give no or very little sugar. (So-called glucose is usually made by a cheap chemical method from maize and has no special value.) Honey in small amounts is best. This should be added to the beverage when it is cool enough to drink, since temperatures over 104°F (40°C) spoil its health-giving properties.

Milk encourages mucus and should therefore only be given diluted to children with throat infections or bronchial catarrh. Small babies, however, must not go without milk for more than three days during the first nine months unless the doctor gives instructions to this effect. Older children with a high temperature often have an aversion to fresh milk but might take it diluted or else might like sour milk, butter milk, yogurt, kefir or similar products. If not, given them fruit juice or plain mineral water.

A child with a temperature needs more liquids. Let him have as much as he wants, but make him sip it slowly. Stewed apple and other cooked fruit may also be given if the illness has not affected the stomach. Sugar should be added in small amounts only, since otherwise there is a danger of diarrhoea or a vitamin deficiency. Fresh fruit is usually preferred and better.

For the main meals try offering a cup of oat or semolina gruel, especially if you can obtain Demeter or other good brands. Rusks, biscuits and bread should also be made from good flour. White wheat or rye flour has no nutritional value. They provide no vitamins for the sick person, indeed they even rob him of his small supply of vitamin B when they have to be digested. So a small amount of good bread with a little butter or good vegetable margarine (no additives!) is better than twice the amount of white bread or biscuits.

The medicine chest

Every household needs a well-stocked medicine chest containing both remedies for illness and first-aid equipment for accidents. It should be placed out of the reach of children and securely locked. A note of the doctor's and chemist's telephone number pinned on the inside of the door is useful. It should contain a book of instructions on first aid for injuries and poisoning. (For the treatment of wounds, see page 198.)

Well-sealed remedies, both liquids and also powders and tablets, can be kept for years. The following list may be used as a guide:

Thermometer
Scissors
Tweezers (large and small)
Feeding cup
Hot water bottle
Safety pins (several sizes)
Leather finger stall
Compresses
Sling
Medicine spoon
Pipette
Kidney bowl
Balloon enema
Enema for children and adults
Cotton wool (large pack)
Bandages
Lint
Gauzes of various sizes
Melolin dressings (non-stick)
W.C.S. Powder (Weleda)
Combudoron (liquid and ointment) (Weleda) for burns

Arnica ointment 10% (Weleda) for sprains

Arnica essence 20% for damp compresses for bruises

Mercurialis ointment 10% for bad bruises and as a drawing ointment (also useful as a nose cream for children!)

Weleda Balsamicum ointment

Calendula essence 20% for damp compresses on open wounds and for rinsing the mouth for bleeding gums

Valerian drops for over-excitement and sleeplessness. Adults 20 drops on a lump of sugar. Babies 4 drops in sugar water

Melissa comp. (Weleda) drops to be taken for stomach upsets and weak spells and used externally for headaches, earaches, etc.

Treatment with water

The general rule is that baths or other applications of cold water should only be made to parts of the body that are sufficiently warm. Also, cold water is only suitable if its use engenders a comforting glow. If the patient does not warm up sufficiently, his circulation can be stimulated by massaging with a brush. If the circulation in the skin improves, the massage can be followed by a quick rub down with cold water.

THE UTENSILS

Containers: A bath or large basin

Wraps and towels: For chest, throat and calf compresses three different cloths are needed. The size will depend on the child's age.

1. The inner cloth is placed wet next to the skin. Rough linen or wild silk are the most suitable materials. The width for throat compresses should be the length of the throat (it must reach up to the ears), and for chest compresses it should reach from under the arms down to the buttocks. Calf compresses must cover the whole calf.

2. The next cloth should also be linen (not cotton). It should be larger above and below than the inner and the outer cloth so that on the one hand the wet inner cloth never protrudes and on the other the woollen outer cloth never touches the skin. Both are uncomfortable for the sick person.

3. The outer cloth is of thick wool or flannel. It should be an inch or two wider than the inner cloth so that no cold air reaches the inner compresses. On the other hand it should be smaller than the middle cloth so that it does not touch the patient's skin.

The cloths should be long enough to go about 1½ times round throat, chest or calf respectively. They may be prepared when the child is well and kept in readiness for when they may be needed. Waterproof material is never necessary.

WASHINGS

This is best done when the child is nice and warm on waking in the morning or when he is really warm in bed in the evening. Fold a coarse hand towel several times and wring out lightly after dipping in cold water. Rub vigorously from the back of the right hand up the outside of the arm to the shoulder and then down again along the inside of the arm to the palm. Do the same with the left arm. If necessary wet the towel again. Wash neck, chest and back with a few strokes. Then starting on top of the right foot wash up the outside of the leg to the buttock and back down the inside to the sole of the foot. Do the same with the other leg and wash vigourously between the legs. The tummy is washed last. The whole operation should take only a few seconds. Put on the night clothes without drying and cover up snugly in bed. If the child does not glow with a cosy warmth at the latest after 10 - 20 minutes, the washing was done too slowly or the room was not warm enough.

Instead of washing the child all over in one sitting, either his upper or lower half can be washed. Usually you would start with his arms and upper part and go on to washing the whole child after a few days.

COMPRESSES

General remarks: Compresses can be applied to throat, arms, chest, loins, legs, calves and feet. The patient must lie in bed during the application.

Damp, hot compresses release cramp and thus relieve pain. The bed and cloths must be well warmed before the compress is applied.

Cold-water compresses 50°-68°F (10-20°C) are used on the one hand to reduce body temperature (the heat is absorbed in the cloths), and on the other to make the patient perspire. To reduce body temperature the inner cloth should be left rather wet. To induce sweating it should be well wrung out, which will cause warmth to build up until the patient breaks into perspiration. When this happens, the compress (which should have no air pockets) is removed. If the compress is too wet or if the water was luke warm instead of cold, it can happen that the child fails to heat it up. In this case it must be removed immediately and the child rubbed with a Turkish towel to warm him. He may need a hot drink of lime-blossom tea as well.

Cold calf compresses are left for 20 minutes and then repeated three to five times at 20 minute intervals. This is usually sufficient to draw the fever down from the head. The patient's discomfort is thus relieved and his face is no longer so hot and red. The compresses should stop when the temperature has been reduced to about 101.3°F (38.5°C), since this will be sufficient to relieve the headache due to pressure of blood in the head.

Cold throat compresses must reach up to the ears and must not be too loose or they will not get warm. As with calf compresses, they can be repeated several times a day.

Hot mustard compresses applied properly and soon enough can relieve pneumonia (and its early stages) dramatically. Stir a heaped dessertspoon of freshly ground mustard (it should have a piercing smell) into a pint of almost boiling water. Dip the inner cloth in this and let it steep. Remove with a wooden spoon and as soon as you can bear to touch it, apply it to the child's chest or to the side affected. Quickly wrap the other

cloths round it. After at most 10 minutes, look to see if
the skin is bright red. If it is, remove the compress
immediately and wash the reddened skin carefully with
lukewarm water. Similarly, remove immediately if the
child cries in pain. Left too long, the compress can burn
the skin. Finally powder the skin (for instance with
Weleda WCS powder).

COLD AND HOT COMPRESSES

Cold compresses should be as cold as possible, never
luke warm. They must never be applied to cold skin.
Hot compresses should be as hot as bearable.

Cold compresses made with several layers of well
wrung cloths reduce bleeding and swelling and relieve
pain where there are injuries, bruises and contusions.
These compresses are not covered with woollen outer
cloths. They are renewed as soon as they start to warm
up, and repeated so long as they bring relief.

Cooling compresses (possibly with a little wine vinegar) can be placed on the heart to calm the patient. A
compress on the back of the neck stems a nose bleed and
also calms the heart of a nervous person.

Wounds, for instance children's cuts and grazes,
should never be washed, even if they are covered in dirt.
Gently pour some water over the place to rinse away the
movable pieces of grit and then cover with dry linen or
gauze. This is then dampened repeatedly but not
removed. The water used for this can contain
Calendula Essence 20% (Weleda or Wala), or Arnica
Essence. A weak salt solution of ¼oz (9g) salt to 2 pints
(1 litre) water will also do if necessary. The wound

needs the greatest possible quiet to enable it to repel the dirt and bacteria.

For burns, Combudoron Lotion (Weleda) is added to the water in accordance with the instructions on the bottle.

Hot compresses are used to relieve painful cramps, for instance gall, stomach and kidney colics. It is a mistake to treat these conditions, which come and go in waves, with an electric blanket or dry hot water bottles. These compresses are also good for menstrual pains in girls and for softening boils, carbuncles and abscesses. They can also be used for bronchitis and pleurisy and inflammation of the joints. Whooping cough, croup and asthma can often be relieved as well.

If hayflowers (flores graminis) are obtainable, make a bag of the required size out of strong material and fill this with the flowers to make a thickness of 5 to 6cm. Place the filled bag in a bowl and pour on enough boiling water to saturate the flowers without making the bag dripping wet. (Wring the bag gently if you put on too much.) If it is well covered up, the bag will hold its warmth for at least an hour. It is very effective and soothing especially for inflamed joints and also for abdominal colics (though for the latter it should not be too heavy).

BATHS

As a rule, late morning and later afternoon are the most suitable times for baths, while the most unsuitable is just before or just after a main meal. Three baths a week is the normal requirement, unless otherwise prescribed.

Warm baths: Temperature between 95 and 98.6°F (35 - 37°C). Bath mixtures made from pine needles, camomile, sloes, rosemary, valerian, kalmus, lavender, sulphur, are used to strengthen or calm the patient or for the treatment of the skin. For duration, see under hot baths.

Hot baths: Temperature between 100.4 and 104°F (38 - 40°C). Baths of which the temperature is gradually raised are very effective in the early stages of colds, bronchitis and flu.

The patient should stay in the warm or hot bath for 10 to 15 minutes. After this, wash or rinse him down with cool water to close the pores opened by the warmth. The bath is followed by three hours in bed.

Schlenz Baths: This method was developed by Frau Maria Schlenz in Innsbruck. It is also described as a warming bath. It can be applied at the beginning of or during acute feverish illnesses such as tonsillitis, flu, incipient pneumonia, bronchitis, pyelonephritis, etc. Professor Lampert of Höxter treated serious infectious diseases such as spotted typhoid, dysentery, and typhoid by this method and I myself have treated soldiers seriously ill with kidney disease in the field hospital in Prague during the war, even when they had high blood pressure. Acute lumbago can be healed in the shortest time and the method is indispensable for the improvement of some chronic complaints and also for the paralysis after polio.

Method: It is important to be very exact. The

patient's bowel is emptied with the help of an enema, after which his temperature is taken. The water temperature at the beginning is made to correspond with this. Stick the end of the thermometer into a piece of cork and let it hang in the water. (Take care: at a temperature of over 107.6°F (42°C) it will burst!)

A decoction of hayflowers (flores graminis) is added to the bath water. For an adult, brew 10-14oz (300-400g) hayflowers in hot water in a bag and let it draw (use less for a child). Pour the decoction into the bath, keeping the bag as a head rest. The patient lies stretched out in the bath with his head on the bag. His neck must be covered by the water which reaches almost to his mouth.

During the first 15 minutes gradually raise the temperature of the water (by using a boiling kettle) to 101.3°F (38.5°C). This serves to open the pores and prepare the patient for the effects of the bath. After this the patient should be warned that he will go through a few minutes of discomfort. His pulse will race and he will feel all the parts that have been affected by the illness. This is the sign that the organism is beginning to react. It may help to scrub the patient's skin with a brush or let him sit up for a moment. This slightly alarming state soon passes and the patient begins to feel comfortable in the bath. The temperature can now gradually be increased to 102°F (39°C). Do not make it any hotter for the patient's first such bath, but maintain this temperature for the rest of the hour which the bath should take. Children often react more quickly and the bath can be ended when they have had beads of sweat on their forehead for some time. But for the full effect the bath should last an hour. Then it is gradually brought to an end. The patient sits up and is then helped to stand up. He is wrapped in a large towel and put straight into bed without drying where he should sweat for another hour well covered up.

After an hour wash the patient with luke warm water to which you can add a little vinegar. Put on dry clothes and put him straight back to bed. Now is the time for a glass of orange juice or other fresh fruit juice. The perspiration will have brought about a considerable loss of vitamin C which must quickly be replaced. Other suitable drinks are rose hip tea, orange or lemon tea sweetened with honey, sandthorn elixir or other Weleda or Wala elixirs.

The Schlenz Bath can also be given as a footbath, for instance for flu, sinusitis, etc. The warmly wrapped patient sits with his feet in a deep bowl or bucket. The hayflower decoction is added and should lead to strong perspiration all over the body, lasting for an hour.

For the second or third bath the water temperature can be increased to 103.1°F (39.5°C) or more, so long as the patient is still comfortable. After a night's sleep he will feel born anew. This bath method has the strongest effect of all water applications. It is particularly suitable when a rapid recovery is required or when an illness drags on for a long time because the patient's forces of resistance are insufficient.

Alternating baths: For children, alternating baths should only be given as foot or arm baths. The feet or arms are warmed first in warm water at 102.2°F (39°C) for 3 to 5 minutes and then immersed in cold water at 46-50°F (8-10°C) for 10 seconds. This is repeated 3 to 5 times, but from the second time onwards only two minutes are necessary for the warm, followed again by 10 seconds immersion in the cold water. The treatment ends with a quick rinse in cold water to close the pores, and the child is then put straight to bed wrapped in a towel (without drying) where he will soon begin to glow with warmth. (Cold water should never be applied to skin that is already cold.)

These baths are particularly suitable for children suffering from cold feet or hands. The series of hot and cold immersions can be done with the feet on one day and with the arms on the next and so on. Such baths are particularly important for youngsters during puberty and in the case of bladder or other abdominal weakness, and also for headache and sleeplessness. Parents should not take it lightly if their children always have cold feet, since this can be the root of a number of serious weaknesses and illnesses.

Regarding daily bathing, see p.87

Poultices

Poultices resemble compresses but do not involve the use of water.

Beeswax poultice: This is used for bronchitis and bad coughs which disturb sleep at night. The beeswax (about 50g for babies and small children) is melted in hot water, on which it floats. A piece of linen is dipped in the melted wax and then quickly placed on chest or back (both if possible) and covered in warm wrappings to keep it hot for as long as possible. The poultice can be left on over night and is very comforting, relieving the coughing.

Similar poultices can also be made with Diphthodoron II (Weleda).

Onion poultice: Sudden pain of the middle ear in babies and small children is relieved within a few minutes by this poultice. Chop a medium-sized onion and put in a muslin bag. Place this on the ear allowing it to overlap on all sides. Cover with a good layer of cotton wool and keep in position with a balaclava helmet. Relief is almost immediate. If it is not, the doctor must be called straight away.

Fenugreek poultice: This works as a drawing paste. The seeds of this plant are used to draw the pus from inflammations (boils, abscesses, etc.). Boil one or two dessertspoons in water to form a thick paste. A layer (¾ inch thick) is placed while as hot as possible on the centre of the boil and left covered with cotton wool till it cools. The treatment is repeated till the pus is discharged, which happens relatively quickly and painlessly, with very little damage to the skin. Lancing can often be avoided in this way.

NOTE 1

The Author's recommendation of certain medicines and other products arises out of his personal experience as a paediatrician and general practitioner and in no way constitutes an advertisement. (Ed.)

NOTE 2

In Britain, decimal potencies are usually indicated as X rather than D. D3 = 3X, which is the equivalent to a dilution of 1 in 1000.

NOTE 3

British 'desert spoon' = American 'soup or table spoon'. British 'table spoon' = American 'serving spoon'.
The British terms are used in this book.

Appendix One

BOTTLES AND TEATS

The glass or plastic baby's bottle is graded showing amounts up to 200g. Larger amounts would be unsuitable and might tempt the mother to give the baby more than 200g at one feed.

The bottle has a rubber cap. Immediately after a meal both are rinsed in cold water and the bottle is left standing full of water. Once a day bottles and caps are washed with a bottle brush in hot water with soda, after which they are rinsed in hot water and left to drip dry. If washing-up liquid is used they must be very thoroughly rinsed with hot water so there is no risk of contaminating the next meal with detergent.

The teat should as closely as possible resemble the nipple. Usually it is already pierced, but if not this can be done with a glowing darning needle. The hole or holes should be just large enough to allow the food to drip through. The drink must not run too easily into the baby's mouth. As with the breast, the baby should have to make a certain effort to obtain the milk.

After every meal the teat is washed thoroughly in cold water to which a little salt may be added. It is then kept in a clean jar with a lid. Both jar and teats must be boiled daily for three minutes. Never touch the end of the teat with the fingers. The smallest remnants of food left in bottle or teat can become the breeding ground for germs which can even endanger life.

UTENSILS FOR BOTTLE FEEDING

1 milk saucepan large enough to boil one pint of milk
1 enamel saucepan (to hold about 2 pints) for cooking Holle baby food
2 - 5 graded baby bottles with rubber caps
1 hair sieve for sieving the baby food
1 - 2 rubber teats with holes
1 bottle brush
1 small saucepan for boiling the teats and the jar in which they are kept
1 glass jar with lid for storing teats
Soda crystals for washing

It is also useful to have:
- a stand for drip-drying the bottles
- a measuring jug (glass) graded up to 250 or even 500g

All these utensils should be used exclusively for the baby's food.

Appendix Three

PREPARING HOLLE BABY FOOD

The gruel

The amount of food to be used is shown on the packet. Mix the food (Holle Oat Flakes, Holle No.1 or Holle No.2) with the amount of water shown and boil for about two minutes, stirring constantly. The gruel is done when it emits a delicious smell of fresh bread. The cooking time can be increased for babies who do not digest too easily. If the baby is not breast fed, it is best to start with oat gruel for the first month and change to Holle No.1 during the second month. This gruel is then used to make the mixtures below.

Half milk, half gruel mixture

Example: Add 100g of the gruel together with two teaspoons of ordinary sugar to 100g of separately boiled milk. The amount for the whole day can be prepared in the morning. After mixing thoroughly it is put into the feeding bottles which are kept in the fridge with their caps on. A bottle is then heated in a water bath when the meal is due.

Two thirds milk, one third gruel mixture

For example 100g is added to 50g gruel. Sweetening and storing of the day's supply as above.

Feeding

Shake the bottle well and then heat up in a water bath. The correct temperature is ascertained by touching your eyelid with the bottle or letting a drop fall on the back of your hand. On no account try sucking the teat. If the baby drinks slowly, the bottle will have to be reheated during the meal, possibly more than once.

Appendix Four

HOW TO MAKE CURD CHEESE

Warm the milk to blood heat and add a spoonful of either sour milk or live yogurt. The bacteria are different, but both result in a souring and thickening of the milk. Allow to stand in a warm place till the milk has thickened. Pour into a muslin or cheese bag and suspend over a bowl for about twelve hours while the whey drains away. The resulting crumbly curds can be used as they are or made smooth by adding fresh cream or milk and whisking gently with a hand whisk.

This is added to the baby's main meal and is the best way of providing his protein needs. For older children and adults it is delicious mixed with finely chopped herbs and eaten on bread or with vegetables. Mixed with chopped fruit or fruit juice it makes a popular dessert.

INDEX